Assessing Mental Health Across Cultures

By
Lena Andary
Yvonne Stolk &
Steven Klimidis

First published in 2003 by
Australian Academic Press Pty. Ltd.
32 Jeays Street
Bowen Hills QLD 4006
Australia
www.australianacademicpress.com.au

National Library of Australia
Cataloguing-in-Publication data:

Andary, Lena.
Assessing mental health across cultures.

Bibliography.
Includes index.
ISBN 1 875378 40 5.

1. Cultural psychiatry. 2. Psychiatry, Transcultural.
I. Stolk, Yvonne, 1943– . II. Klimidis, Steven. III. Title.

616.89

Cover and text design by Andrea Rinarelli of Australian Academic Press, Brisbane.
Typeset in Adobe Garamond by Australian Academic Press, Brisbane.
Printed by Watson Ferguson & Company, Brisbane.

Contents

List of Information Boxes

Preface

While a wide array of literature is available on various aspects of crosscultural mental health assessment, this book is designed to meet an acknowledged need for a publication that draws together this literature, and elaborates the clinical implications of the impact of culture on key aspects of mental health assessment. Our principal audience, mental health practitioners and students entering professional careers in mental health, are provided with a theoretical and clinical guide to cultural and linguistic issues likely to be encountered in their work with clients from a culture different from their own. This work arose out of the clinical experience of the authors and their experience of developing and delivering a new training program in crosscultural psychiatric assessment to numerous mental health practitioners in Victoria, Australia, over a period of 12 months. The training program was developed in response to expressed needs for such training by mental health practitioners. The book followed requests for a reference publication to enable the practitioners to consolidate their learning.

The book is organised to constitute an integrated whole. While each chapter addresses discrete issues that have been identified by mental health professionals as relevant to clinical practice, each chapter builds on information and ideas developed in the preceding chapter. The aim of this step-wise integrative process is to provide a comprehensive framework for approaching a crosscultural assessment. The chapters that follow do not endeavour to resolve major theoretical debates in the field of crosscultural mental health (such as the relative contributions of biology and culture to differing manifestations of mental illness across cultures). Rather, crosscultural differences that clinicians are likely to encounter in daily practice are discussed, and illustrated with case examples, to enable clinicians to avoid misdiagnosis and to plan appropriate treatment.

Chapter 1, Issues and Dilemmas in Diagnosis Across Cultures, provides the theoretical underpinnings for the clinical chapters that follow. The cultural assumptions underlying diagnoses in the DSM-IV are introduced, with the aim of alerting clinicians to those theoretical issues that may impact on daily clinical practice. A case study is used to highlight the complexity of the clinical and psychosocial issues involved in crosscultural assessment, raising the clinical implications to be explored in greater detail in the chapters that follow. Chapter 1 closes with an introduction to the cultural formulation, a framework that is applied to case examples in the later clinical chapters.

Chapter 2, Cultural Values, the Sense of Self and Psychiatric Assessment, examines the nature of culture and highlights values as a key aspect of culture with significant implications for clinical practice. Comparisons are drawn between the cultural values and assumptions about the self that are brought to the clinical interview by the Western clinician and the non-Western client.

Case examples are provided to illustrate the influence that values can have on the clinical relationship, on the assumptions that the client and the clinician make about the nature of normality, and on the effectiveness of treatment. Strategies are included to raise clinicians' awareness of their own and their clients' values framework.

Chapter 3, Expression and Communication of Distress Across Cultures, explores differences in the regulation, expression and interpretation of affect and mood across cultures to search for an answer to the question, "Does depression exist across cultures?" The chapter examines assumptions about emotion that underlie Western culture and Western mental health practice and questions whether these assumptions have universal application. Common assumptions about somatic symptoms are explored in the context of the connection between the mind and the body in Western and non-Western cultures.

Chapter 4, Issues in Translating Mental Health Terms Across Cultures, explores the potential for miscommunication in translating mental health terminology across cultural and linguistic barriers. Guidelines are provided for working effectively with interpreters. The cultural fairness of psychological tests and measures is also scrutinised in this chapter.

Chapter 5, Explanatory Models of Illness, investigates the influence of crosscultural beliefs and explanatory models of illness on illness definition, help-seeking and acceptance of treatment. An emphasis is placed on developing an understanding of explanatory models, and how they may be elicited by the clinician in a crosscultural situation.

In **Chapter 6**, Crosscultural Beliefs About Illness, a range of crosscultural explanations of illness are discussed and two major belief systems, or worldviews, namely the Evil Eye and Spirit Possession, are examined in some detail to draw out their implications for mental illness and treatment. Principles are provided for distinguishing culturally sanctioned behaviour and ideas from psychopathology.

The purpose of **Chapter 7**, Negotiating Explanatory Models, is to explore the process of negotiating discrepancies in explanatory models between the clinician and client that may lead to rejection of treatment. The chapter then integrates the clinical issues that have been raised throughout the book. A transcript of an interview illustrates the process of negotiating explanatory models, while highlighting the cultural issues relevant to the various aspects of the case. To illustrate how the cultural features of a case can be communicated to other clinicians, the case study described in the interview transcript is then reported in a culturally sensitive clinical formulation in the final part of the chapter.

Where possible, this book provides strategies for overcoming barriers to effective crosscultural assessment. The authors do not pretend, however, to have all the answers or to provide a "cookbook" to guide clinicians through every aspect of crosscultural clinical communication and comprehension. Crosscultural mental health assessments need to be informed by an awareness of one's own cultural values, assumptions and beliefs, and the points at which these may result in misunderstanding. The present work provides some guidelines for reducing such misunderstandings. Other key ingredients of successful crosscultural psychiatric assessment are time and a genuine interest in understanding the person being assessed.

Acknowledgements

The authors gratefully acknowledge the support and encouragement of Associate Professor I.H. Minas, Director of the Centre for International Mental Health and of the Victorian Transcultural Psychiatry Unit, and other staff of the Unit. The important part played by NorthWestern Mental Health in supporting the development and implementation of the training program in Crosscultural Psychiatric Assessment is also gratefully acknowledged. Guy Coffey, Senior Clinical Psychologist, and Thuy Dinh, Bilingual Case Manager and Psychologist, both of South West Area Mental Health Service, are thanked for their valuable contribution to development of the strategies for negotiating explanatory models and for commentary on chapter 5. We particularly wish to express our appreciation to Lorraine Stokes, Librarian of the Australian Transcultural Mental Health Network, for providing information and guidance in matters of publication. The eight Area Mental Health Services that agreed to participate in the training in 1999 are thanked for releasing staff from Crisis Assessment and Treatment Teams and other programs. The participating services were The Alfred, Central East, Inner West, Mid West, North West, Outer East, South West and St Vincent's Area Mental Health Services. Special thanks go to the clinicians who attended the training and participated in vigorous debate about the issues, thereby contributing their perspectives to this book.

The Authors

Lena Andary is a clinical psychologist who teaches for the Graduate Diploma in Community Mental Health at Melbourne University. Lena has worked with mental health services since 1992, including acute psychiatric inpatient units, crisis assessment and treatment teams and outpatient clinics. At the time of writing her position was as Ethnic Mental Health Consultant, which involved assisting mental health services in the Eastern Region and Inner South of Melbourne to improve their responsiveness to consumers from culturally and linguistically diverse backgrounds. Lena's work has included the development and implementation of policy, research, training and education of mental health clinicians, and community development. Her particular area of interest has been the clinical implications of working with persons from linguistically and culturally diverse backgrounds in terms of assessment, understanding and treatment. Lena is also a member of the Australian Centre for Psychoanalysis and has completed the Centre's 4-year course.

Yvonne Stolk is a clinical psychologist who worked for 8 years in community and inpatient mental health settings. Since 1997 she has been employed by NorthWestern Mental Health as an Ethnic Mental Health Consultant, working with mental health services in the Western Region of Melbourne to increase sensitivity of staff to clients of cultural and linguistic diversity and to improve access to services by ethnic communities. The training program that formed the basis of this book was developed collaboratively with her co-authors in response to training needs identified as part of research Yvonne is undertaking for her PhD with the Centre for International Mental Health, Department of Psychiatry, University of Melbourne. She has also worked as a research psychologist participating in evaluation and epidemiological studies of mental health, including a 2-year prospective study of newly-arrived Indo-Chinese refugees. She was a contributing author to *The Price of Freedom: Young Indochinese Refugees in Australia*, edited by Krupinski and Burrows in 1986. In addition to a number of journal articles and research reports Yvonne co-authored *Not the Marrying Kind: Single Women in Australia*, in 1983, which was based on research for her Master's thesis.

Steven Klimidis was awarded his PhD at the Australian National University in the field of clinical psychology in 1989. In the past decade he has worked as a clinical psychologist in private practice and within public health agencies. He has acted as consultant to numerous projects ranging from mental health promotion, service models development and clinical services evaluation. He has authored research papers, book chapters and reports in areas as diversified as psychiatric epidemiology, the phenomenology of psychoses, evaluation of health care services and transcultural mental health. Steven's research has more recently concentrated on how culture might be best conceptualised as it affects the nature of psychological distress, the help-seeking process and the therapeutic relationship. Currently he is the Assistant Director and Coordinator of Research of the Victorian Transcultural Psychiatry Unit and holds the position of Associate Professor in the Centre for International Mental Health, Department of Psychiatry, University of Melbourne.

The authors would like it to be known that Lena Andary and Yvonne Stolk are equal primary authors of this work.

Chapter 1

Issues and Dilemmas in Diagnosis Across Cultures

Key Points

▶ Crosscultural applicability of Western syndromes

▶ The concept of culture-bound syndromes

▶ WHO studies of depression and schizophrenia

▶ Culture and the DSM-IV

▶ Elements of cultural assessment

"... the basic concepts of psychiatry reflect the culture and history of Western Europe-influenced societies**"**

(Griffith, 1996, p. 27)

I n multicultural communities mental health clinicians regularly face the challenges of conducting crosscultural psychiatric assessments. Regardless of their professional discipline and the type of mental health service they provide, mental health practitioners routinely use assessment skills, either implicitly or explicitly, when they see new clients and when they work with ongoing clients. New clients are assessed to determine whether or not the person is suffering from a mental illness. If they are, the assessment endeavours to establish the diagnosis and recommends appropriate interventions. If, as a result of the assessment, it is concluded that a client does not have a mental illness then they are discharged or referred to a more relevant service. For continuing clients, assessment is an ongoing task, as the clinician routinely assesses the client's mental state and psychosocial adjustment to monitor whether the client is at risk or whether they have recovered.

In these processes mental health professionals implicitly apply a conceptual diagnostic framework to the client. This framework usually derives from the most influential diagnostic classification systems of the West, such as the *Diagnostic and Statistical Manual of Mental Disorders* (*DSM-IV;* American

Psychiatric Association [APA], 1994) or the *International Statistical Classification of Diseases and Related Health Problems* (*ICD-10;* World Health Organization [WHO], 1992). In this book we focus on the DSM-IV but will be referring to Western[1] diagnostic systems in general. Although, in the course of their work, mental health professionals such as social workers, psychiatric nurses or occupational therapists may not, themselves, make formal psychiatric diagnoses, they will often carry an internalised diagnostic template based on systems such as the DSM. This is difficult to shed since most of their mental health training, most peer communications regarding client psychiatric problems, and most of the research published carries this framework. This means that the behaviour, speech and demeanour of the client are likely to be matched against DSM or ICD criteria. To demonstrate this, consider what diagnostic options come to mind when faced with the following "symptoms". Loss of appetite: *depression?* Anergia/passivity: *depression, schizophrenia?* Belief that spirits possess the person: *delusional disorder, schizophrenia?* Avoidance of eye contact: *depression, social phobia?* The behaviour of a client who touches the clinician and asks personal questions may be interpreted as *intrusive* or *disinhibited.* These interpretations of "psychopathology" are rooted in Western diagnostic systems. Much of what currently is known about psychopathology, and about what are considered to be specific categories of mental disorder, is drawn from research that is conducted with Western notions of what constitutes normality and abnormality and what constitutes disorders such as schizophrenia and major depression. It is virtually impossible for the clinical thinking of mental health clinicians not to be structured by a Western psychiatric framework, as clinical training, until recently, has ignored alternative perspectives for understanding and responding to mental disorders (Myers Wohlford, Guzman, & Echemendia, 1991; Sue et al., 1982; Westermeyer, 1985).

There is now a growing literature on crosscultural issues in mental health. Training courses are more likely to address crosscultural issues in mental health and a number of cultural features have been included in the DSM-IV. These cultural features will be discussed later in this chapter. Unfortunately, neither the literature nor the DSM-IV provide clear directions to mental health practitioners on how to conduct an effective crosscultural mental state examination, and how to incorporate cultural factors into case formulations, diagnoses and treatment planning. In this book we attempt to compensate for these absences.

To familiarise ourselves directly with some of the crosscultural issues faced by mental health professionals, let's consider the case of a 24-year-old

---

1 *West, Western cultures*: Includes North America, Western Europe, Britain, Ireland and Australia. These are countries with cultures predominantly committed to the empirical scientific method as a source of knowledge (Gaines, 1982). Alternative terms for Western are "Euro-American", and somewhat less accurately, "Anglo-Saxon".

Nigerian man.[2] He was referred to a community mental health service by his general medical practitioner who wrote:

> Dear Clinician,
>
> Thank you for seeing Samuel whom I have been seeing for 2 months with complaints of feelings of heat in his head, and the sensation that worms or ants are crawling in his head. In addition he complains of visual blurring and pain in his eyes. Investigations have failed to find evidence of a parasitic disease or other diagnosable physical disorder. He has been assessed by an optician but does not require spectacles. I am referring him to you for a psychiatric assessment.
>
> Yours faithfully,
>
> Dr English

What follows is a formulation of Samuel's case made by the assessing clinician. While reading the report, the reader may wish to consider what provisional diagnosis or diagnoses might apply to this client:

A Case Example: Samuel

Presenting Symptoms

Samuel is a 24-year-old single Nigerian man who is currently on sick leave from his job as an apprentice electrician. He was referred by his GP because of persistent feelings of heat in his head and the sensation of insects crawling in his head. He complains that he started developing severe headaches when he commenced studying for his electrical apprenticeship 6 months ago. The pain of the headache seemed to burn him on the head and his head felt unusually heavy. He said his headache developed in such a way that he seemed to be tired of life. After some time he developed the feeling that something was walking or crawling about in the centre of his head. He became unable to read because he felt that words had lost their meaning and because of visual blurring and pain in his eyes. During classes he feels unable to take in what is taught and when he talks he feels the words don't come from his brain but only from his mouth. Glare and any attempt to read appears to exacerbate the headache. Only sleep seems to alleviate the condition, but he often has difficulty falling asleep. He also reports having lost his appetite. On direct questioning he admitted feeling sad, and sometimes wonders whether life is worth living with the persistence of this condition. He denied using alcohol or illicit drugs. He wondered whether one of his neighbours might be a witch and had caused his problems by casting an evil spell on him.

Current Circumstances

Samuel arrived from Nigeria 9 months ago, with his mother and two younger sisters and they are sharing a house with another

---

2 Case compiled from Guinness (1992a, 1992b), Harris (1981) and Prince (1985).

family. His mother is unemployed and his sisters are in high school so he is the breadwinner for the family. He speaks English moderately well. He is studying for his apprenticeship at Western Institute of Tertiary Education and is apprenticed to Smith Electricians. He feels pressured to do well at his studies by his mother and they frequently argue. He is particularly worried that his symptoms will interfere with his performance in exams, which are in two weeks time.

Past History of Symptoms and Treatment
He began to experience symptoms shortly after starting his studies. His symptoms impaired his concentration at work and he sought medical advice because his employer became impatient with his poor progress and absences on sick leave. He takes Panadol regularly, but this has little effect on his symptoms.

Family and Personal History
Samuel attended 4 years of high school in Nigeria where his academic performance was average. His family ran a small farm and was poor, but they were committed to giving Samuel a good education. Family conflict occurred frequently as his father drank alcohol heavily. The family fled Nigeria after his father and brother were killed in cross-fire during fighting between opposing political parties. Samuel has made only a few friends since arriving in Australia. Other than his father's alcoholism, Samuel is not aware of any history of mental illness in his family.

Mental State Examination
Samuel was a tall thin young man who was casually and neatly dressed and groomed. He made poor eye contact but spoke readily about his problems. He appeared at times anxious and perplexed at the effect of his symptoms and at other times despondent and despairing about his situation in relation to his family, and his study and work prospects. He showed a limited range of affect and his mood appeared somewhat lowered. He acknowledged he had wondered whether life was worth living but had no active plans to commit suicide. There was no evidence of formal thought disorder or of auditory or visual hallucinations, but he was preoccupied with his many somatic symptoms and delusions and notions of having been bewitched. Samuel was oriented in time, place and person, and his memory appeared to be intact.

Formulation and Diagnosis
Samuel is a 24-year-old single Nigerian man who arrived in Australia 9 months ago with his mother and two younger sisters. Samuel is studying and working as an apprentice and is the only breadwinner in the family as his father and brother were killed in Nigeria. He was referred by his GP with unusual somatic symptoms and concerns that he might be suicidal. At assessment he admitted to 6 months of lowered mood, impaired concentration,

sleep and appetite and to suicidal thoughts. He describes headaches, ocular pain and visual blurring, feelings of depersonalisation, cranial sensory hallucinations and delusions that he has been bewitched. His symptoms have caused him to take frequent sick leave. He denies substance abuse.

Differential Diagnosis

Major depressive disorder; generalised anxiety disorder; undifferentiated somatoform disorder; mood disorder with psychotic features; delusional disorder: mixed type (somatic and persecutory); schizophrenia; cognitive disorder with associated anxiety and depression.

To justify the differential diagnoses mentioned above, Figure 1.1 shows how Samuel's symptoms might fit each diagnosis. Following discussion of Samuel's case in the clinical team meeting, neuropsychological testing was carried out to rule out cognitive disorder due to organic causes. These tests indicated normal cognitive functioning, but impaired concentration. The neuropsychologist felt that impaired concentration was possibly due to depression and anxiety. Treatment with Diazepam somewhat improved Samuel's ability to study, but he still complained of the heaviness and crawling sensations in his head. The addition of antidepressant medication appeared to make little difference to his condition. Samuel dropped out of treatment after 3 months, but his case manager subsequently heard that he had sought treatment from a traditional healer who had provided traditional treatment to ward off an evil spell that Samuel felt he was under. After this, Samuel had successfully completed his exams and had become involved in an African volunteer welfare group in his spare time.

Culture-bound Disorders

One diagnosis not considered by the clinical team was the African syndrome called "brain fag", which is listed in the Glossary of Culture-Bound Syndromes in Appendix I of DSM-IV. As described in the DSM-IV, brain fag is:

> A condition experienced by high school or university students in response to the challenges of schooling. Symptoms include difficulties in concentrating, remembering, and thinking. Students often state that their brains are 'fatigued.' Additional somatic symptoms are usually centred around the head and neck and include pain, pressure or tightness, blurring of vision, heat or burning … (APA, 1994, p. 846).

Virtually all of these symptoms were experienced by Samuel, although his sensations of something crawling in his head are not included in the DSM-IV's account of brain fag. This is surprising as quite a number of research studies in Africa have reported this symptom as a common feature of brain

FIGURE I.I

The relationship between diagnoses and symptoms for the Samuel case example.

Diagnosis	Symptoms
Major depressive disorder	• Sadness, head feels heavy • Fatigue, tired of life • Disturbed sleep and appetite • Impaired concentration • Impaired occupational functioning • Suicidal ideation
Generalised anxiety disorder	• Uncontrollable anxiety about work, study and family • Fatigue • Irritability • Impaired sleep • Impaired concentration • Impaired occupational functioning
Undifferentiated somatoform disorder	• Multiple physical complaints (headache, crawling and heat in head, fatigue, blurring and pain in eyes, loss of appetite) which can't be explained by known general medical condition • Impaired occupational functioning
Mood disorder: with mood-congruent psychotic features	• Symptoms as for major depression and, • Somatic delusions of crawling and heat in the head
Delusional disorder: mixed type (somatic/persecutory)	• Non-bizarre somatic delusions (head infested with parasites)
Schizophrenia	• Delusions of control (witchcraft) • Somatic/tactile delusions • Deterioration in functioning
Cognitive disorder	• Headache • Visual blurring and pain, susceptible to glare • Impaired concentration • Somatic illusions • Aphasia (words have lost meaning, unable to take in what he reads and what is taught) • Impaired memory (unable to learn or recall previously learned information) • Deterioration in functioning

fag (Ebigbo, 1982; Prince, 1985). The fate of this symptom within the DSM will be revealed shortly, but first it is necessary to define what culture-bound syndromes are and to consider why they are not accorded formal status as disorders within the main classification system of the DSM-IV (Littlewood, 1996). According to the DSM-IV:

> The term culture-bound syndrome denotes recurrent, locality-specific patterns of aberrant behaviour and troubling experience that may or may not be linked to a specific DSM-IV diagnostic category. Many of these patterns are indigenously considered to be 'illnesses,' or at least afflictions and most have local names (APA, 1994, p. 844).

Some authors in the field suggest that the expectations and constraints of culture tend to influence how distress is expressed and how it is perceived (Rogler, 1993). The influences of culture, therefore, may organise symptoms into particular types of disorders. Culture-bound syndromes may be seen as an example of differing configurations of symptoms, or as idioms of distress, which are sets of symptoms that cluster together in ways that differ from syndromes in other cultures (Rogler, 1993). Alarcon (1995) has suggested that the term "culturally defined patterns of distress" (p. 456) may be more meaningful than the term "culture-bound syndrome".

The distinction between culture-bound syndromes and other syndromes described in the DSM system is not at all clear. The DSM-IV explains that culture-bound syndromes are not included among the main DSM categories because of their "localised" occurrence. While disorders that correspond with DSM categories can be found throughout the world "culture-bound syndromes are generally limited to specific societies or culture areas and are localised, folk diagnostic categories" (APA, 1994, p. 844). The American Psychiatric Association is therefore asserting that the main DSM categories can be found universally (that is, across all cultures) and that universality is a precondition for official DSM status. As we discuss below, the assumption of universality does not hold even for the main DSM categories of illness (e.g., anorexia nervosa). In addition, the assertion that culture-bound syndromes are "folk diagnostic categories" implies they have a lower status than "professional" labels of distress. Some psychiatrists believe that if culture-bound syndromes were admitted as "official" disorders this would result in "an unnecessary proliferation of psychiatric labels" (Prince, 1985, p. 201), suggesting that culture-bound syndromes are redundant (i.e., contain no new information) within the existing descriptive classification system.

However, culture-bound syndromes, including brain fag, *are* considered to be pathological conditions in their local culture (Littlewood, 1996). By separating culture-bound syndromes and giving them restricted status, the DSM-IV creates the risk that these conditions will be dismissed by clinicians as marginal or irrelevant (Hughes, 1996). If DSM-IV categories are the only categories officially considered to be disorders, what is a clinician to record as a diagnosis for Samuel on official forms that require a DSM-IV diagnosis and/or an ICD-10 numerical diagnostic code? DSM-IV's response to this question is that conditions such as brain fag should be "translated" into any matching forms of pathology that can be found within the main categories of disorder. Thus brain fag should be interpreted by the clinician as "an idiom of distress [that resembles] certain [forms of] anxiety, depressive, and somatoform disorders" (APA, 1994, p. 846). Clinicians wanting to record a diagnosis can sort culture-bound "aberrant behaviour" that forms part of "a single folk category" into several DSM categories (APA, 1994, p. 844). Ostensibly this appears to involve no more than a mere translation of cultural distress into the DSM framework, but much may be lost in this process. The vexed question arises whether such translations provide a valid description of the client's distress and, most importantly, whether the new category or categories have any personal validity or meaning for the client.

The differential diagnosis exercise carried out above for Samuel's symptom presentation is an example of what can occur if we were to use the recommendations of the DSM-IV in translating brain fag into DSM-IV categories, including anxiety, depressive and somatoform disorders. The problem with this disaggregation of Samuel's symptoms into Western disorders is that *each* diagnosis requires something to be left out (and may also assume the presence of some symptoms that are not part of the client's experience). None of the suggested differential diagnoses fits Samuel's presentation as well as brain fag. Perhaps the closest category is that of major depressive disorder, where the DSM-IV Specific Culture Features state that:

> Culturally distinctive experiences (e.g., fear of being hexed or bewitched, feelings of 'heat in the head' or crawling sensations of worms or ants …) must be distinguished from actual hallucinations or delusions that may be part of a major depressive episode, with psychotic features (APA, 1994, p. 324).

As this quotation shows, symptoms of crawling sensations have not been overlooked by the DSM-IV; they have been extracted from the brain fag syndrome to be included in the culture features for major depressive episode. But this account does not acknowledge that these symptoms actually form part of a common and meaningful African syndrome (Kirmayer, Young & Hayton, 1995). By dismembering this African idiom of distress the DSM-IV ignores the fact that local syndromes are embedded in systems of local meaning (Lewis-Fernandez & Kleinman, 1995). Should the clinician work on the basis of an "artificial" (DSM) syndrome that poorly fits the experience of the client, or should the clinician try to capture the client's experience by yielding towards a diagnosis that is meaningful within the client's culture?

Culture plays a critical part in the meaning that patients give to their disorder and in the treatments that they seek. Samuel did not understand his

Box 1.1

Social Background to Brain Fag

Research into brain fag demonstrates the role the social, cultural, economic and political context plays in the onset and manifestations of the disorder. It also highlights the risks of misinterpretation that can result from the use of Western measures of psychopathology in non-Western cultures.

Prince (1985) and Guinness (1992a, 1992b) found that brain fag tends to be experienced by African students in primary and high schools, and particularly by those studying for tertiary entrance exams. Education is an important issue in many African countries because it is the means for economic advancement and increasing one's social status, both for the student and the student's family. Therefore there are high expectations for achievement both from the student and from the family. The social origins of the disorder are demonstrated by a relationship between the symptoms and a range of psychosocial factors. Symptoms of brain fag are more likely to be reported by students from poor families, where the parents have a low level of education. There is also likely to be conflict in the family, perhaps associated with alcoholism. Guinness (1992b) also reported that students with brain fag were more likely to have been raised by their grandmother because their parents were migrant labourers. Grandmothers may have multiple grandchildren to care for so that the nutritional and/or personal needs of any one child may be overlooked.

A study of brain fag by Guinness (1992a, 1992b) compared students' spontaneous descriptions of their health with their responses to the Self-Reporting Questionnaire (SRQ) to determine whether the brain fag syndrome resembled Western diagnostic syndromes. While somatic symptoms were the most commonly reported symptoms, both spontaneously and on the SRQ, anxiety and depressive symptoms as elicited by the SRQ were found to have different meanings in the Swazi context than intended. Some items included in the SRQ to assess affect seemed to be simply culturally irrelevant (Guinness, 1992a). SRQ questions designed to screen for psychosis also were found to be of dubious validity. Students who endorsed SRQ questions such as "interference with thinking" feared that others were envious of them and might bewitch them. One student reported, for example, that "someone took my books to bewitch them, to put spells in the pages to enter my eyes as I read" (Guinness, 1992a, p. 47). Guinness (1992a) states that these are certainly not psychotic symptoms but "spiritual" symptoms associated with problems in concentrating and remembering. In other words, the brain fag syndrome did not neatly fit any one Western syndrome. ■

problem as one of depression (and in fact it cannot be fully understood in any of the terms of the main DSM categories of disorder). To offer him treatment for depression would not be consistent with his understanding of his problem. He appears to have recovered in response to treatment by a traditional healer, a treatment that is consistent with Samuel's understanding that he had been bewitched (Harris, 1981). That is, often the "folk" diagnosis is more meaningful because it provides treatment options that are likely to be effective in resolving the problem. Ignoring the clinical reality of the client means that such critical options will be ignored and opportunity for effective treatment lost. Samuel's case provides an illustration of a number of important issues that can arise in crosscultural clinical work. The client and the mental health professional have brought to the clinical interaction different cultural values, different assumptions about the expression and meaning of distress and differences in their beliefs, "explanatory models", and treatment expectations. Each of these issues will be examined in more detail in the chapters that follow.

As mentioned earlier, the main DSM disorders are not necessarily universal, and the claim that they are reflects a certain ethnocentrism[3] built into the DSM. The DSM-IV for example includes anorexia nervosa as one of its core disorders rather than as a culture-bound disorder. Transcultural psychiatrists have argued that if there is to be a separate section for culture-bound disorders, then anorexia nervosa should be included as a Euro-American culture-bound syndrome (Kleinman, 1996; Levine & Gaw 1995; Prince, 1985). It is acknowledged in the DSM-IV's Specific Culture Features for anorexia nervosa that the syndrome is most common in Western countries and Japan, where being slim has come to signify beauty and desirability (Kleinman, 1996). Although this Western syndrome is not universal, in this instance it has not been consigned to Appendix I of the DSM-IV. Ignoring the evidence in stating that "little systematic work has examined prevalence [of anorexia nervosa] in other cultures" (APA, 1994, p. 543), the DSM-IV implies that universality of anorexia nervosa is merely pending.

In insisting that its categories are universally applicable the DSM-IV fails to recognise that all psychiatric categories are to some extent culturally constructed (Littlewood, 1996). Is it impossible then to take a universal approach to psychiatric diagnosis? Should each culture have its own culturally specific diagnostic system? To answer these questions it is necessary to examine whether an "etic" or an "emic" approach is to be preferred in crosscultural clinical practice and research. The next section examines these two approaches.

---

3 *Ethnocentrism*: "Ethnocentricity is the inherent tendency to view one's own culture as the standard against which others are judged" (Senior & Bhopal, 1994, p. 329).

Universality or Cultural Relativism?

After all, diagnosticians can be trained so that they are consistent but wrong (Kleinman, 1988, p. 11).

Clinicians, in everyday practice, face the same dilemma as crosscultural researchers. Should they apply a so-called universal classification system to a non-Western client, or should they side-step this diagnostic taxonomy and attempt to form an understanding of the illness experience from the client's perspective? This is the choice between an etic or an emic perspective.

An etic approach is generally used by Western researchers with an empiricist scientific background who enter other cultures searching for universals in human behaviour. In this process, external illness models are imposed onto local illness categories (Smith & Bond, 1993). Epidemiological studies, such as those of the World Health Organization conducted in the last few decades (to be described later), have used an etic approach. They applied "standard" instruments developed in the West to identify the nature and prevalence of mental disorders in various population groups across the world. It is more rare to find non-Western researchers attempting to establish the prevalence of concepts of mental illness from their own culture in a Western population (Littlewood & Lipsedge, 1989; Obeyesekere, 1985). An example of such a (rare) study is Prince's (1985) comparative study of brain fag in Canada. Prince was not a non-Western researcher, but a Canadian psychiatrist who had worked in Nigeria where he became aware of the brain fag syndrome. After studying its manifestations in Africa, he surveyed Montreal high school students to determine whether they suffered brain fag symptoms, such as burning or crawling sensations, or feelings that words didn't make sense when reading. Not surprisingly, the proportion of students complaining of such experiences was very low in Canada (Prince, 1985). The reason his findings are not surprising is that he was looking for symptoms of a disorder that had no relevance in Canadian culture. Conversely, how confident can a Western-trained mental health worker be in applying Western categories of disorder to non-Western cultures?

Prince's study is an excellent example of a type of problem identified by Kleinman (1988), which he termed a "category fallacy". A category fallacy occurs when the diagnostic categories of one culture are applied to people in another culture, where those categories lack coherence, have no pathological salience and the relevance of those categories has not been established (Kleinman, 1988). To apply DSM-IV diagnostic categories, which have been developed from studies of Euro-American middle-class patients, onto people in non-Western cultures (such as Samuel) involves a category fallacy (Kleinman, 1988). Provocatively, Patel and Winston (1994) suggest that, until validated in non-Western countries, Western psychiatric categories might be best classed as "folk" categories of Euro-American thought.

Universality by Default?

An example of category fallacy on a grand scale is provided by the World Health Organization's (WHO) international studies of depression and schizophrenia, which were conducted in the 1960s, 70s, and 80s. WHO researchers entered other cultures looking only for phenomena that fitted predetermined Western diagnostic categories, without establishing whether those categories were meaningful or relevant to people in those cultures. The WHO findings are often cited as demonstrating the universality of the major Western mental disorders, thereby justifying the use of Western diagnostic categories across cultures. The WHO studies have also helped to shape the taxonomy of the DSM-IV and to justify its claim that the DSM's main forms of disorder categories are universally applicable (Fabrega, 1989). But the WHO research precluded the possibility of finding syndromes that differed from Western syndromes. A mental health professional risks making the same error when applying DSM-IV categories to the problems presented by a non-Western client. By applying a Western clinical template, those experiences of the client that do not fit may not be elicited, may be overlooked or minimised, raising the likelihood of misdiagnosis.

It needs to be acknowledged that even within the constraints imposed by the etic method, crosscultural differences were found by the WHO studies. However, these differences (described in boxes 1.2 and 1.3) were minimised in the reports of results, while crosscultural similarities were highlighted. Nevertheless, the findings of the WHO studies did throw some light on the nature of possible differences in the onset, manifestation and course of mental illness across cultures.

The WHO Study of Depression

The WHO study of depression investigated whether "a typical diagnostic stereotype of depression" could be found across cultures (Jablensky, Sartorius, Gulbinat & Ernberg, 1981, p. 371). Canada and Switzerland (so-called "developed" countries), Iran and Japan (so-called "developing" countries) were assumed to represent a sufficient sample of international cultures (Jablensky et al., 1981). Case detection methods focused on a "checklist" of a series of symptoms that were generated from Western conceptions of what constitutes depression. Not surprisingly then, reports of their findings emphasised that the same "core" of depressive symptoms could be found in the majority of patients across cultures. Nevertheless, some crosscultural differences in the manifestations of depression were observed, although dismissed as "relatively minor" (Sartorius et al., 1980, p. 748). These included higher levels of the experience of guilt and self-reproach in developed countries, while somatic symptoms were reported more frequently in the developing countries (Sartorius et al., 1980). Crosscultural differences in levels of suicidal ideation showed a more complex pattern (see Box 1.2 for details).

Box 1.2

Crosscultural Similarities and Differences
Found in the WHO Study of Depression

The core of symptoms of depression found universally in 76–100% of patients included sadness, anxiety, anergia, anhedonia, impaired concentration and feelings of worthlessness.

Details of the crosscultural differences were as follows: people in all four countries reported guilt experiences, but guilt and self-reproach were more common in developed countries, with 68% of patients in Switzerland endorsing such experiences, 58% in Canada, 48% in Tokyo, 41% in Nagasaki and 32% in Iran (Sartorius et al., 1980). Somatic symptoms, including lack of appetite, loss of weight, loss of libido, and constipation, were more common in "developing" than "developed" countries. Fifty-seven per cent of patients in Teheran reported such symptoms, 32% in Switzerland and 27% in Canada (other centres not reported) (Jablensky et al., 1981). Suicidal ideas were reported by 59% of all patients, but the numbers varied from 41% in Tokyo, 46% in Teheran to 70% in Montreal and Nagasaki (Sartorius et al., 1980, Jablensky et al., 1981). ■

The WHO study of Schizophrenia

One of the key aims of the 10-country WHO Study of Determinants of Outcomes of Severe Mental Illness was to determine the rate of schizophrenia across cultures (Jablensky et al., 1992). As in the study of depression, "standard" instruments and narrow inclusion criteria enabled the WHO to conclude that a universally consistent syndrome of a narrowly defined florid schizophrenia could be found at a rate that showed little variation across cultures. In actual fact there was substantial variation in the prevalence of this syndrome across nations; the highest rate (of 1.4 per 10,000 population in England) was double that of the lowest rate (of 0.7 in Denmark). A broader syndrome showed significantly different rates of disorder across cultures, ranging from 1.6 per 10,000 in Denmark to 4.2 in rural India.

Again cultural differences in manifestations of schizophrenia were de-emphasised in reporting results. Nevertheless, it was found that patients from developing countries were more likely to have an acute onset and to experience only a single psychotic episode followed by complete remission. Those in developed countries were more likely to show a gradual onset and a chronic disorder (Jablensky et al., 1992). The most common diagnoses were acute schizophrenia in developing countries, but paranoid schizophrenia in developed countries. Catatonic schizophrenia was more commonly diagnosed in developing than in developed countries. The symptomatic profile also differed: the most common symptom reported by patients in developing

Box 1.3

Crosscultural Similarities and Differences
Found in the WHO Study of Schizophrenia

The WHO study found that patients with acute onsets of schizophrenia had the most favourable outcome and those with gradual onsets the least favourable outcomes. Acute onsets were most common in developing countries, with 51% of patients showing an acute onset, compared with 28% in developed countries. Conversely, a gradual onset was shown by 30% of patients in developing countries, but by 52% in developed countries. Earlier findings suggesting improved outcome in developing countries were supported: 37% of patients from developing countries experienced only a single psychotic episode followed by complete remission in the 2 years following the study, compared with 16% of patients from developed countries. Patients from developed countries, on the other hand, were more likely to have had psychotic episodes for 76–100% of the 2-year follow-up period.

Acute schizophrenia was the most common diagnosis in developing countries, being diagnosed in 40% of cases, compared with only 10% in developed countries. Paranoid schizophrenia was the most common diagnosis in developed countries, being diagnosed in 34% of patients and in 23% in developing countries. Even though patients with paranoid schizophrenia generally had a worse outcome than those with acute schizophrenia, in developing countries, even those with paranoid schizophrenia had a better outcome than patients with acute schizophrenia in developed countries. Catatonic schizophrenia was diagnosed more often in developing (10%) than in developed countries (1%). The most common symptoms (reported by more than 30% of cases) showed some similarities across cultures, but auditory hallucinations were among the common symptoms reported by patients in developing countries (52%) but not in developed countries. Depressed mood was a common symptom for patients in developed countries (56%), but not for patients from developing countries (Jablensky et al., 1992). ■

countries was auditory hallucinations, while patients from developed countries were more likely to report depressed mood.

The Same Disorders?

Is it reasonable to assert that the disorders identified by the WHO studies in non-Western cultures are the same disorders as those found in Western cultures? The constraints of Western measures only enabled differences in emphasis to be revealed: higher or lower population rates, a greater frequency of one symptom than another, a longer or shorter course. But when rates, onset, symptoms, course and recovery are shown to differ in studies not designed to reveal these differences, it seems reasonable to question whether the disorders are the same. Etic studies, however, are not designed to answer such questions; this requires an emic approach.

When cultural differences are found (e.g., wide international variation in suicide rates) the etic researcher fails to investigate the local meaning of symptoms in order to obtain an understanding of the factors that contribute to symptom variations. At best, variations from the "universal" may be cast into the "culture-bound" basket. Failure to investigate the meaning of a symptom may also occur in a clinical setting when the DSM-IV is applied unthinkingly across cultures. The emic approach attempts to examine how pathology emerges from within the cultural millieu, how it is labelled and responded to by members of the culture.

As demonstrated by the WHO studies, Western syndromes can be found with high reliability across cultures, but this does not mean that the syndromes identified are valid. Clinicians can be trained so that they agree (i.e., show high reliability) on what they observe (or are asked to observe and record in a research study), but that does not mean that the client has a disorder consistent with a Western diagnostic category, or even that the client has a mental disorder at all (Fabrega, 1989; Kleinman, 1988).

Clinical Implications

Professionals working in mental health services, who are not aware of the ethnocentric assumptions of the DSM-IV, will find, like the WHO researchers, that they will obtain confirmation of DSM's diagnostic categories when they ask a standardised set of clinical assessment questions. What may be missed by this process is the individual's culturally-shaped experience of distress. What the WHO studies, and studies using an emic approach (see next section), have shown is that the symptom manifestations and course of mental illness do vary across cultures. If classifications are applied that have no relevance in the culture of the person being assessed it is likely that the thing being measured will be empty of meaning (Obeyesekere, 1985). This may result in inappropriate treatment or loss of contact with the client, as occurred in the case of Samuel.

Integrating Culture into Psychiatric Assessment

If current Western conceptions of mental illness are not universally applicable, how are mental disorders to be assessed and recognised across cultural boundaries, and how can we know whether the categories we apply are crossculturally valid? To obtain an authentic understanding of the illness experiences of another culture, and to avoid risks of crosscultural misunderstandings and misdiagnosis, an emic approach should be used (Smith & Bond, 1993; Strongman & Strongman, 1996). This means that local illness categories should be identified and studied over time within a culture in groups of similar patients (Patel & Winston, 1994). Locally developed measures should be used to study the characteristics, course, treatment and outcome of a disorder. This process is not unlike the ethnographic method used by anthropologists, who develop long-term relationships with small numbers of people in a particular culture to study a social phenomenon in depth (Kleinman, 1988). Once an emic perspective has been used to develop diagnostic criteria that are locally valid, these illness categories can be used in etic studies to compare categories from various cultures and to identify common and possibly universal features. This combination of emic and etic approaches is most likely to clarify how mental disorders differ across cultures and how they are similar (Kleinman, 1988).

The emic (or ethnographic) methods used by anthropological psychiatrists have had a major influence on mainstream psychiatry, ultimately leading to the acknowledgement of the role of culture in the DSM-IV. Examples include studies of idioms of distress in China (Kleinman, 1980, 1988), in Iran (Good & Good, 1982), in Puerto Ricans (Guarnaccia, Rubio-Stipec & Canino, 1989) and in Native Americans (Manson, Shore & Bloom, 1985).

At the level of mental health clinical practice, a crosscultural clinical interview can similarly be viewed as an opportunity to conduct an emic study of a client's illness experience. Later in this book we discuss how a clinician can obtain an in-depth understanding of the client's idiom of distress using such an approach. We term this an individual-cultural approach. Diagnostic categories provide a shorthand means of communicating complex processes between clinicians and guide the choice of treatment. But diagnostic categories give little or no consideration to personal, social and cultural issues, which are central for the person to whom the categories are applied. The individual-cultural approach is a process that involves working beyond the framework of Western diagnostic labels. The benefit is that this approach can facilitate a relationship of trust between the client and clinician and can help in framing a culturally sensitive strategy to treatment. If clinical practice (and official paperwork) require that the client's experiences be fitted into a Western diagnostic framework, then the clinician has at least acquired an understanding of the client that extends beyond these boundaries and can influence treatment strategy.

Culture in the DSM-IV

In this section we explain the endeavors made to have cultural factors included in the DSM, the cultural features that are included, and the shortcomings of the final "concessions" that were made. It is worth remembering that the development of the various editions of the DSM represents a process of consensus among "expert" clinicians and researchers from a vast variety of areas of expertise. As a process based on agreement it should (theoretically) accept the relativity of its final content. For example, homosexuality is no longer a mental disorder within the DSM system, but it was in the first edition. Similarly, posttraumatic stress disorder was not a diagnosis in the DSM system until the 1980 edition of the manual, but since its incorporation into the DSM a whole mental health industry has developed around this diagnostic category. Similarly, given that the content of the DSM is constructed through a process of agreement between experts, it is open to the influence of political processes that determine who is an expert and what is admissible, relevant, necessary or peripheral clinical knowledge. This means, in plain terms, that the lower status afforded to cultural influences on psychopathology, as communicated by the DSM-IV, represents an opinion held by numbers of currently powerful and dominating professionals within American psychiatry. This does not mean their opinion is wrong (or right), but it does represent a perspective on psychiatric phenomena.

A second point to remember is that despite the "hard-won" ground in introducing cultural factors into the DSM, there remains a major gap in the implementation of cultural analysis in day-to-day clinical practice. In 1999, 5 years after the publication of the DSM-IV, a survey by the authors of 88 clinicians, the majority of whom were working in mental health crisis teams where clinical assessment is their primary task, revealed that only 10% were aware of any of the cultural features included in the DSM-IV (Stolk, 2002). We will return to this issue later. For now we examine the cultural content of the DSM-IV.

Until the fourth edition of the DSM the question of the crosscultural applicability of DSM diagnostic categories rated no more than a cursory mention within the covers of earlier editions (Alarcon, 1995; Kleinman, 1996). Not until the publication of DSM-III-R (APA, 1987) was a brief caution included in the Introduction. This cautionary note stated that since the DSM was developed in the United States, difficulties might occur in applying its diagnostic categories across cultures (Stein, 1993). In response to critiques from many transcultural psychiatrists and anthropologists (Fabrega, 1987; Good, 1993; Kleinman, 1988; Lock, 1987), the American Psychiatric Association acknowledged the relevance of cultural factors to psychiatric diagnosis and established a Task Force to work on the issues of culture in relation to the forthcoming DSM-IV (Alarcon, 1995; Kleinman, 1996; Mezzich, Kleinman, Fabrega & Parron, 1996). This Task Force enabled the American Psychiatric Association to state that, "The involvement of many international experts ensured that DSM-IV had available the widest pool of information and would be applicable across cultures" (APA, 1994, p. xv). The Task Force made recommendations for the incorporation of cultural issues in all aspects of the Diagnostic Manual but, to the dismay of the Task Force members, much of their advice was rejected or modified (Good, 1996b; Lewis-Fernandez & Kleinman, 1995). In practice the cultural features that were included were as follows:

- One page on ethnic and cultural considerations in the introduction drawing attention to the potential, when using the DSM-IV in culturally diverse populations, to "incorrectly judge as psychopathology those normal variations in behaviour, belief or experience that are particular to the individual's culture" (APA, 1994, p. xxiv).

- Specific Culture Features in the text for a number of diagnostic criteria, which describe "cultural variations in the clinical presentations of these disorders" (APA, 1994, p. xxiv).

- An Outline for a Cultural Formulation "designed to assist the clinician in systematically evaluating and reporting the impact of the individual's cultural context" (APA, 1994, p. xxiv) presented in Appendix I.

- A Glossary of Culture-Bound Syndromes, also in Appendix I.

While these inclusions in the DSM-IV represent important gains, relatively little of this cultural information is considered in the DSM-IV as crucial for reaching a diagnosis (Kleinman, 1996). For example, culturally-influenced symptoms described in Specific Culture Features are not integrated as inclusion and exclusion criteria for the diagnosis of a disorder (Kleinman, 1996; Good, 1996a). This was illustrated by the case of Samuel, whose symptoms of "crawling sensations of worms or ants" in the head *are* described in the Culture Features for Major Depressive Episode, but are *not* included in the critical criteria for making a diagnosis of depression.

The relegation of the Cultural Formulation and the Culture-Bound Syndromes to the 9th Appendix on page 843 of the DSM-IV is likely to mean that few clinicians will be aware of their existence, as suggested by our survey described above. This lack of awareness of the Cultural Formulation by mental health professionals is unfortunate, as it contains, in our view, among the most valuable of the crosscultural information included in the DSM-IV. The Outline for a Cultural Formulation provides a tool that prompts clinicians to undertake a:

> ... systematic review of the individual's cultural background, the role of the cultural context in the expression and evaluation of symptoms and dysfunction, and the effect that cultural differences may have on the relationship between the individual and the clinician (APA, 1994, p. 843).

A modified version of the Cultural Formulation will be presented at the end of this chapter to introduce this framework for conducting cross-clinical assessments.

Cultural Shortcomings of the DSM-IV

We have already alluded to a number of the cultural shortcomings of the DSM-IV, such as the failure to integrate cultural issues into its conceptual framework in order to make it "a truly international classification" of mental disorders (Stein, 1993, p. 323). Other recommendations made by the Task Force on Culture and the DSM-IV that were not accepted were the inclusion of:

- case illustrations to accompany the Cultural Formulation

- the term "and Idioms of Distress" added to the title "Glossary of Culture-Bound Syndromes"

- two categories of illness: dissociative trance disorder and mixed anxiety-depressive disorder

- anorexia nervosa, chronic fatigue syndrome and dissociative identity disorder as Western culture-bound syndromes (Lewis-Fernandez & Kleinman, 1995).

According to Lewis-Fernandez and Kleinman (1995), the final set of exclusions and modifications meant that the effort of the Task Force to enhance the cultural validity of the DSM-IV had failed. Despite the crosscultural failings of DSM-IV, clinicians employed in mental health services are implicitly or explicitly required to use the DSM-IV's diagnostic categories in documentation and in making decisions about the disposition of their clients. While using its classification system, clinicians need to be aware of the many culturally derived assumptions that underlie DSM criteria.

Underlying Assumptions of the DSM-IV

> Implicit in the entire structure of the diagnostic process [are] particular cultural commitments — normative views of the person and societal judgements about … "antisocial" behavior — basic categories and distinctions (e.g., thought vs. affect, somatic vs. affective) (Good, 1996b, p. 348).

Fundamental to the lack of crosscultural validity of the DSM-IV are ethnocentric assumptions about the nature of human activity, the self, emotions, the mind and body, society, normality and pathology. In this section some of these assumptions will be introduced and then explored in greater detail in subsequent chapters.

An individualist sense of self. Criteria for mental health in DSM-IV imply that the person should have a stable, individualist sense of self, defined independently of, or separately from, others. Those who do not strive for autonomy, those who are "dependent" on a group, and those who reject personal responsibility are viewed as psychologically immature or inadequate. These assumptions are examined further in chapter 2.

Psychopathology resides inside the individual. It is assumed that psychopathology resides in the individual rather than in the interaction between the individual, other people, physical, historical and spiritual realities. Assumptions regarding the location of personal experience are examined further in chapter 2 and chapter 3.

Disorders can be differentiated into discrete categories. Despite a statement in the Introduction of the DSM-IV to the contrary (p. xxii), the categorical nature of DSM-IV diagnoses implies that disorders can be clearly differentiated. As demonstrated with Samuel's case, a focus on categories shifts attention away from levels of distress and an insistence on strict diagnostic boundaries "force[s] the diagnostic dismemberment of popular illnesses that combine features" of several DSM categories (Good, 1993; Lewis-Fernandez & Kleinman, 1995, p. 437). Aspects of these assumptions are explored further in chapter 3.

Mental disorders are universal and biologically caused. As prefigured in the WHO studies, the categories and disorders identified in the DSM-IV are assumed to be universal (Kleinman, 1996). It is assumed that evidence about a disorder in a Euro-American population "is generalisable to all humans, because one is learning about basic human (that is, biological) processes" (Good, 1996b, p. 349). The search for universally similar illness presentations across vastly different cultures implies biological underpinnings to mental illness (Kleinman, 1988; Lin, 1996). This search for universality is misguided, as known biological illnesses are themselves by no means universal. For example, conditions such as hypertension, diabetes mellitus and Tay-Sachs disease all vary substantially across different cultures due to both genetic and environmental reasons (Lin, 1996; Patel & Winston, 1994; Westermeyer, 1985). The role of cultural and social factors in the onset and course of a disorder are often discounted (Lewis-Fernandez & Kleinman, 1995). Some of the biological assumptions underpinning Western psychiatry are further examined in chapter 3.

The whole world speaks a direct translation of English. In claiming to "be applicable across cultures" and to have "wide international acceptance" (APA, 1994, p. xv–xxiv), the DSM-IV implicitly assumes either that the whole world speaks English, or that its terminology can be readily translated into languages other than English without loss or distortion of meaning and without changes in connotation (Wierzbicka, 1992). This assumption is inextricably linked with assumptions that categories that describe and, in turn order experience, are equivalent across cultures. These assumptions are further examined in chapters 3 and 4.

Principles of Cultural Assessment

When conducting a crosscultural psychiatric assessment, a number of topics should be incorporated into the assessment interview to obtain a comprehensive understanding of the person within their social and cultural context. The main questions the clinician should bear in mind are:

1. What is the cultural identity of the client?

2. What is the cultural presentation and what are the cultural explanations of the illness?

3. What cultural factors are related to the psychosocial environment and to levels of functioning?

4. What are the cultural elements of the relationship between the client and the clinician?

5. What is the overall cultural assessment and formulation for diagnosis and care (DSM-IV, Appendix I)?

The following sections define the specific domains of information relevant to these key questions. Further detail expanding on each of the questions will be provided in the remaining chapters of this book. The domains described below are based loosely on the Outline for a Cultural Formulation in DSM-IV's Appendix I (APA, 1994), Minas (1996a) and the authors' own clinical and research experiences.

Cultural Identity

- *Cultural group membership.* What is the client's preferred ethnic identity, gender and religion?

- *Language.* Which language does the client speak at home? Which language do they prefer to speak? How proficiently do they speak English? Is an interpreter required? Are they multilingual?

- *Cultural factors in development.* For example, is the client a refugee? Have they had war experiences? Do they experience racism? What are the gender-based expectations in their culture?

- *Acculturation.*[4] What is the extent of involvement with the culture of origin and with the host culture?

Cultural Presentation and Explanation of Illness

- *Predominant idioms of distress and local illness categories.* Does the client or their family communicate the problem through a "local" idiom of distress?

- *Meaning and severity of symptoms in relation to cultural norms of the reference group.* For example, is a sick role for the disorder culturally sanctioned? What is the degree of stigma associated with the disorder?

- *Explanatory models of the individual and his family.* What does the person and their family call the problem? What do they think causes it? And what treatment do they think is needed?

- *Help-seeking experiences and plans.* In the context of the explanatory model, what traditional and other help has already been sought? And what other treatments are being contemplated?

Cultural Factors Related to Psychosocial Environment and Levels of Functioning

- *Social stressors related to culture.* For example, is there intergenerational value conflict in the family? Are there culturally-based role expectations?

---

4 Acculturation may be defined as a process of cultural change that occurs (in an individual or cultural group) with close, continuous contact between two culturally distinct groups (Minas et al., 1996, p. 23).

- *Available social supports.* Is the family, or extended family, normally relied on in the culture of origin present in Australia? Are available social supports culturally sensitive? What is the role of religion in the life of the individual?

- *With respect to cultural norms, what is the person's level of functioning and disability?*

Migration History

- *What is the country of birth of the person?*

- *In what year did they arrive in Australia?*

- *What motivated them to migrate?* Were they a refugee from war or persecution? Were they seeking family reunion? Were they seeking better economic conditions or better educational opportunities for themselves or their children?

- *Is there history of pre-migration trauma?*

- *Circumstances of migration.* Did they travel directly to Australia or via a third country and refugee camps?

- *Which significant people were left behind?*

- *What have been the major benefits of migration?* For example, safety, family reunion, economic.

- *What were the major losses associated with migration?* Has there been a loss of contact with the family, death of family members during flight, loss of occupational status or unemployment?

Cultural Elements of the Relationship Between the Person and the Clinician

- *Adequacy of communication.* How do differences in culture, social status and language influence communication between the client and clinician and interfere with eliciting symptoms? Are there cultural taboos regarding gender in the clinical relationship?

- *Forms of deference.* How does the client expect to be addressed, and how do they expect to address the clinician? Are there cultural conventions regarding interpersonal communications?

- *Power relationship.* Does the client expect a relationship of equality or deference with the clinician?

- *Confidence and trust.* Is the client familiar with the nature of mental health services and professionals? Have there been past experiences that might have caused distrust of government organisations? Do they believe that what is offered is relevant to their problem?

Overall Cultural Assessment for Diagnosis and Care

- A clear statement concerning what cultural factors are relevant to this client at this time, how such factors may influence onset, persistence of the illness or recovery, help-seeking, and the course and outcome of the illness.

Further detail elaborating on each of these areas of the cultural assessment will emerge throughout this book. An example of a complete cultural formulation will be provided in the last part of this book.

Chapter 2

Cultural Values, the Sense of Self and Psychiatric Assessment

---

Key Points

▶ Defining and raising awareness of culture and values

▶ Key value dimensions with implications for assessment

▶ Differences in values across cultures

▶ Cultural values of Western psychiatry

▶ Cultural conceptions of the self: clinical examples

This chapter takes a more clinical perspective on issues of culture, focusing on problems that can arise in the crosscultural clinical encounter and in the process of implementing treatment. The emphasis is on the relationship between the clinician and client and the role played in that relationship by culture, cultural values, and cultural constructions of the self.

Alarcon (1995) suggested that culture is a multifaceted concept, finding more than 200 definitions of the term, each showing variation according to the context in which it was used. For the purpose of this chapter the essential elements of some of these definitions have been condensed (see box 2.1, Definitions of Culture) and selected for discussion because they are relevant to the context of mental health assessment. "Culture" is used in different ways to mean different things and in any one instance the concept may be ill-defined. What does a clinician mean when they say, "The difficulties in this family are cultural; the family is enmeshed"? Statements of this kind suggest that the term culture is used to summarise personal attributes of the members of a group.

There is an implication that such cultural attributes are stable and that, by extension, culture is stable. However, reference to our definitions suggests that culture is a process that is constantly defined and redefined through people's interactions. What is not so evident in this statement is that the person is drawing a cultural contrast, and in the process, making a value-laden judgement from a particular cultural vantage point. Without conscious effort this may not be avoidable. We are not generally conscious of the influence of culture in our lives; it tends to be taken for granted, like the air we breathe. Culture is not like a coat that can be taken off and discarded. Often it is only when we are confronted by a different culture that we become aware of our own. This is true for us and for people from other cultures. We tend to use our own culture as the standard and judge other cultures (or individuals) by that standard (Triandis, 1990).

Culture involves daily assumptions about shared meaning that allow people to communicate, to live and work together, and to interpret each other's behaviour and motives. A society's major institutions, for example, health and education systems, reflect and express culture as do sex roles, professional roles, and social class. We may assume that what goes on in our culture is "natural" and "correct" and that our own "ingroup" customs, norms, roles and values are universally valid. As a consequence of this there is a tendency to favour the ingroup and to experience hostility towards "outgroups" (Triandis, 1990).

Culture is not the same as ethnicity. Senior and Bhopal (1994) endorse the view that ethnic groups "are characterised by a sense of belonging or group identity" (p. 328). Ethnicity is self-defined, and in both research and clinical settings people should be asked to voluntarily nominate their own ethnicity (Senior & Bhopal, 1994). An example of self-defined ethnicity from the authors' own case files occurred during a clinical case discussion in a mental health setting when one of the patients presented was said to be Palestinian. Another clinician protested that the patient could not be Palestinian because there is no such country as Palestine. The team concluded that it was important to respect a person's own definition of ethnicity. The importance of self-definition is also highlighted in the plight of other groups such as the Macedonians who protest against their redefinition as Yugoslav or Greek, or the Kosovars who, at the time of the political crisis (1998–1999), were identified as Albanians despite multiple generations having lived in Kosovo. All were examples of re-definitions of ethnic identity due to political processes and may not have corresponded to an individual's self-perceived identity. In a different setting, where there was no political duress, a United States study found that one-third of people nominated a different ethnic group when asked to assign themselves to an ethnic group in two consecutive years (McKenzie & Crowcroft, 1994). Ethnic identity may therefore be dynamic.

Box 2.1

Definitions of Culture

- Culture is a process arising out of shared ethnicity, religion, beliefs, language, knowledge, values, meanings and rules, which enable members of a given society to communicate, live, work, anticipate and interpret each other's behaviours and motives.

- Culture is to be found not in the mind of the isolated individual, but in the connections between members of groups such as families, work settings, networks and whole communities.

- Culture provides meaning to social interactions through a pervasive set of symbols that are reciprocally built up out of everyday experiences of social life. Through all these elements, culture patterns ways of thinking, feeling and reacting. Consequently, culture shapes and guides the behaviours and the expectations of individuals. Cultural rules govern the expression of emotion and expectations regarding the role of the individual in society.

- Cultural rules govern illness behaviour — we learn "approved" ways of being ill.

- Culture "programs" behaviour as systems of symbols and meanings are internalised by children during socialisation. Cultural codes are submerged beneath consciousness; only when we are deprived of culture do we become aware of it.

- Culture is heterogeneous. There are layers of culture: gender, generation, social class, work roles. Culture is composed of many voices contesting and negotiating moral issues: about what is at stake, and how these things are to be achieved.

- Culture provides a template that reduces the complexity of the world to manageable simplicity, providing a map that predetermines what to see, believe and value, and how to interpret perceptions, respond and think about oneself.

These definitions were drawn from the following references, Alarcon (1995), Corin (1996), Draguns (1989a), Hofstede (1980), Kleinman, Eisenberg and Good (1978), Kluckhohn (1951), Lewis-Fernandez and Kleinman (1995), Kleinman, (1996), Mezzich, Kleinman, Farega and Parron (1996). ∎

Aspects of culture include:

- language
- values
- religion
- knowledge and beliefs
- rules
- meanings.

These differing aspects of culture can be used to distinguish one group from another. Each area will be explored further in this book; however, at this point in the discussion, values are of particular interest as they are one of the key means of defining differences between cultures and have direct implications for clinical work.

Values

Values represent what is considered important or desirable in a culture and are embodied in the principles and moral standards by which people live. These principles and standards differ across cultures. As values influence the actions and judgements of individuals and social groups they may be seen as motivating forces, underpinning much of human striving (Brown, 1993; Hofstede, 1991; Schwartz & Bilsky, 1987). Values are often a reflection of a culture's religious, spiritual and worldly beliefs. This can be seen in the moral injunctions of the Ten Commandments of Christianity, the Eightfold Noble Path of Buddhism, and in the precepts of Confucianism, which are discussed in further detail in chapter 6.

In the following sections of this chapter we will explore in further detail how a culture's values impact on conceptions of mental illness and on the clinical relationship. Because values influence expectations regarding the nature of "normal" behaviour, any sort of behaviour that falls outside the boundaries of these norms may be judged as "abnormal". While cultural values influence conceptions regarding what is normal and abnormal behaviour, in turn these conceptions affect the way that mental illness is manifested or expressed in different cultures. Within these culturally-based conceptions of normal and abnormal are implicit assumptions regarding the nature of the person or "self", about how individuals should relate to each other, and about how emotions are to be experienced, interpreted, regulated and expressed. Each of these value-based issues impact upon the relationship that a client and their family has with a mental health worker.

When Values Clash

As mentioned earlier, we only become aware of our own culture when we are confronted with a different culture. When the clinician said at the start of this chapter that the family was "enmeshed" there was an implicit, culturally-based assumption that adult individuals in a family should be independent, and that there should be a clear difference and space between family members (i.e., they should be differentiated, not enmeshed). These values, however, do not prevail across all cultures. The way that family members relate to each other and to those outside the family is culturally determined. Consider the following additional examples:

- Speaking about a client of Mediterranean background, a clinician said, *"He's 30 and still lives at home. It's cultural. He's a real mummy's boy."* Implicit in this statement are value assumptions regarding the appropriate age of independence and the ending of family responsibility towards offspring.

- Another clinician introduced himself to a Vietnamese client: *"Hi, Duc. I'm Andrew Jones, just call me Andy."* This greeting contains implicit assumptions regarding appropriate gestures of deference and respect.

- Clinical staff have asked, *"Why is the family such an issue for some cultural groups?"* Underlying this question is an implicit expectation that the nature of the relationship between the individual and the family in some Western societies should prevail universally, and surprise that it does not.

These examples demonstrate that many assumptions are made about the nature of the person, or self, and the about the values that are held by clients and clinicians — all of which affect clinical practice.

The Hofstede Model

One way of understanding the nature of the value differences in these situations is Hofstede's (1980) values framework. After analysing data collected from 50 countries (see Box 2.2, Hofstede's International Study of Values), Hofstede proposed four crosscultural value dimensions:

- Individualism–Collectivism
- Power Distance
- Uncertainty Avoidance
- Masculinity–Femininity

For the purpose of this book only individualism–collectivism and power distance will be discussed, as these dimensions appear to have the most direct implications for crosscultural assessment of mental health.

Box 2.2

Hofstede's International Study of Values

Hofstede (1980, 1991) studied differences and similarities in national patterns of culture. IBM employees in 50 countries were surveyed using a questionnaire designed to investigate "employees' personal values related to the work situation" (Hofstede, 1980, 1991, p. 251). He surveyed 88,000 employees in the late 1960s and early 1970s, obtaining 117,000 questionnaires. From these data he identified four value dimensions on which all cultures could be placed. Hofstede argued that values are among the building blocks of cultures, contributing to the stability of cultural patterns across generations.

Hofstede acknowledged criticisms of his extrapolation of IBM employees' values to those of a nation. IBM employees are generally considered to be middle class and are not representative samples of national populations (Hofstede, 1991). He argued that cross-national comparisons don't require representative samples, but they do need to be "functionally equivalent" (p. 251). By being well-matched, "the only thing that can account for systematic and consistent differences between national groups within such a homogeneous multinational population is nationality itself" (p. 252).

Hofstede's empirically established dimensions confirmed three issues that previous studies had identified from the literature on national character and personality. These issues included: 1) relation to authority; 2) conception of self, including conceptions of masculinity and femininity; and 3) primary conflicts and ways of dealing with them, including the expression of emotion (Hofstede, 1980).

Hofstede's model is only one way of conceptualising values and has its limitations. Draguns (1989b) expresses reservations about Hofstede's equation of nations with cultures. While this equation causes few problems where states are culturally homogeneous and speak the same language (e.g., Japan, Austria), it is problematic in pluralistic nations such as Canada or India. This nation/culture equation obscures large sources of within-country cultural variation.

Because Hofstede developed his measures of values from a Western, etic perspective, the Chinese Culture Connection (1987) developed an emic scale of basic values for Chinese people that was translated and administered to students in 22 countries around the world. Although a quite different scale was used, three of the four dimensions found by Hofstede were replicated: collectivism (called integration); high power distance (called moral discipline); and masculinity (called human-heartedness). The uncertainty avoidance dimension was not replicated, but another dimension called Confucian work dynamism (labelled long-term versus short-term orientation by Hofstede, 1991, p. 164) was identified. Values defining this factor included persistence; ordering of relationships by status and observing this order; thrift; having a sense of shame;

personal steadiness and stability; protecting your "face"; respect for tradition; and reciprocation of greetings, favours and gifts (Chinese Culture
Connection, 1987; Hofstede, 1991). ∎

Figure 2.1 shows a country's score on the individualism–collectivism
dimension on the vertical axis and its score on the power distance dimension
on the horizontal axis. A high score on the individualism–collectivism dimension means that that country tends to have individualist values, while a low
score means that a country's values tend to be collectivist. Low scores on the
power distance dimension indicate that a country tends to have low power
distance and high scores indicate that it is high on power distance. The figure
shows that individualism–collectivism and power distance are inversely related
— high power distance countries tend to be more collectivist, while low power

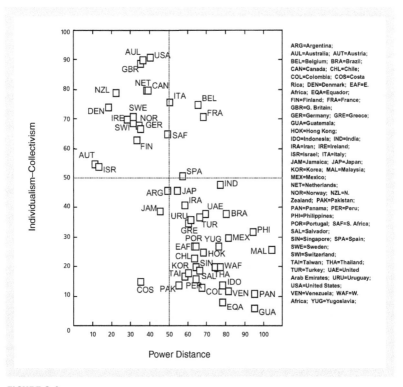

FIGURE 2.1

The relationship between Power Distance and Individualism–Collectivism across different nations (based on
Hofstede, 1991, p. 54).

distance countries are more likely to be individualist (Hofstede, 1991). For example, Australia, the United States and Great Britain scored high on individualism but relatively low on power distance, while Thailand and Hong Kong scored low on the individualism–collectivism dimension (and therefore collectivist) and high on power distance.

The Individualism–Collectivism Dimension

The individualism–collectivism dimension describes the relationship between the individual and the collectives that prevail in a given society (Hofstede, 1980). Individualism refers to societies where the ties between individuals are loose — everyone is expected to look after him or herself and his or her immediate family. Collectivism, on the other hand, pertains to societies where people from birth onwards are integrated into strong, cohesive ingroups, which throughout life continue to protect them in exchange for unquestioning loyalty (Hofstede, 1991).

Individualist and Collectivist Concepts of Self:
Independence and Interdependence

Whether a culture has collectivist or individualist values has a strong bearing on its concept of the self, because a culture's value orientation pervades all aspects of life, including approaches to child-rearing (Hofstede, 1991; Smith & Bond, 1993). Markus and Kitayama (1991) compare differences in the way that the "self" is defined by people from Western and Eastern societies. They distinguish between an independent sense of self, which tends to be associated with individualist cultures, and an interdependent sense of self, which is more likely to be associated with collectivist cultures (Markus & Kitayama, 1991). In individualist Western cultures identity is focused on the "I", the development of an independent sense of worth, of personal efficacy and of self-determination. Self-actualisation and autonomy are the developmental goals for an individual from an individualist culture. Children are expected to become self-reliant and independent by differentiating from their parents and leaving the family home as soon as they have enough education to stand on their own feet (Hofstede, 1991). To be independent means that one's behaviour is interpreted (made meaningful) by reference to one's own internal thoughts and feelings, not by reference to the thoughts, feelings and actions of others. The person is viewed as the integrated centre of awareness, emotion, judgement and action set in a social environment of other such self-contained beings. "To be a self is … to be [an agent] a source of activities, a creator of actions, plans, chains of thought, speculations" (Gauld & Shotter, 1977, p. 171). While the independent self is responsive to the social environment, social responsiveness is primarily an avenue for the expression of the differentiated and independent self (Markus & Kitayama, 1991).

In contrast, in collectivist Eastern cultures, where an interdependent self is said to prevail, identity is defined through reference to the person's social context, emphasising consideration of others (Markus & Kitayama, 1991). There is a tendency for children to learn to think in terms of "we", and personal worth and sense of self-efficacy is measured by the degree to which the person complements the goals of others. Outcomes and achievements are negotiated in collaboration with the social sphere. Mature interdependence is seen as the ideal of personal development for the person from a collectivist culture, by which is meant that the individual promotes shared responsibility, social harmony and consensus in society. The self is most meaningful and complete within the context of appropriate social relationships. The person is less differentiated from and does not seek to be separate from others. This is well captured in the Hindu saying that "Hell is separation from others" (Markus & Kitayama, 1991, p. 228). Markus, Mullaly and Kitayama (1997) illustrate the independent and interdependent senses of self by using the metaphors of a computer and a plant. In Western cultures the self can be compared to a computer, which carries its software internally and is invariant in its action no matter where it operates. In contrast, the Eastern self is likened to a plant, which depends fundamentally upon its natural environment for its development and survival. This means that in Western culture the "person-environment", "self-society", "inside-outside" distinctions are more definite than in Eastern culture.

A culture's attitude towards the idea of self is often evident in forms of personal address (Khai, 1994). For example, in Vietnamese there are no words for "I" and "you". Instead, others and the self are addressed in terms of relationships, such as "uncle" and "little sister". In this situation a person is defined not on the basis of individual attributes, but upon their position and role within the family. An "older brother" has certain responsibilities in common with all "older brothers". These terms are also applied to people who do not literally occupy that relationship to the individual, but they denote relative terms of respect. For example, all older persons are addressed as "aunt" or "uncle". When speaking of oneself, one's own name is used, but only in association with the relationship to another person (e.g., "little sister Anh"). This demonstrates that this conception of the self only has meaning in relation to others.

It is important to appreciate that the descriptions we provide may not characterise any single individual, but represent general tendencies within cultures (Hofstede, 1991). This point is demonstrated in Figure 2.2, which shows findings from a study we conducted that compared the individualism–collectivism scores of medical students from Malaysia (a country scoring high on collectivism) and Australia (a country scoring high on individualism) (Klimidis & Minas, 1998). It is clear that many Malaysian students obtained scores that placed them at the individualist end of the dimension, while many Australian students obtained scores that placed them at the collectivist end. The individualist and collectivist selves are idealised, categorical extremes along a continuum that are used to illustrate certain tendencies.

FIGURE 2.2

Distribution of Collectivism scores for medical students (Klimidis & Mimas, 1998).

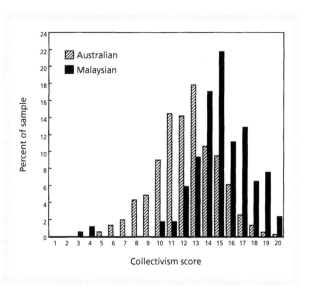

Although the self is referenced with respect to others in collectivist cultures, this does not mean that equal consideration is given to all other people. People from collectivist cultures are not simply more social or altruistic than those from individualist cultures. What may be motivating these behaviours are the relationships between ingroups and outgroups.

Ingroups and Outgroups in Collectivist Cultures

In collectivist cultures an important distinction is made between members of ingroups and outgroups (Triandis, 1990). The most common and fundamental ingroup is the family, whether this is defined as the extended or the immediate family. (Typically in traditional collectivist cultures the family is the extended family, including aunts, uncles, and cousins.)

Fundamental differences exist in collectivist cultures between behaviour towards the ingroup and the outgroup. Speaking one's mind is valued and encouraged in individualist cultures, regardless of whether this is directed to ingroup or outgroup members. In collectivist cultures the value of speaking one's mind depends on whether what is said contributes to the preservation of harmony of the ingroup. Thus, while one may readily contribute opinion that maintains ingroup harmony, communication is more tempered if it is likely to disturb ingroup harmony. The need to "fit in" and not disturb ingroup harmony as opposed to the ideal of differentiation is well captured by the following Eastern proverbs, "Mature rice bends to the ground", and "The nail that stands out gets hammered down" (Markus, Mullaly & Kitayama, 1997).

In collectivist cultures harmony is more important than assertiveness and the rights of the individual. Harmony in the social unit is paramount in collectivist societies and, in the interests of harmony, the individual learns the importance of attending to the needs of others while subjugating their own interests (Markus & Kitayama, 1991). The needs of others may take on such importance that the other's goals are experienced as one's own goals. Because of the expectation of reciprocity:

> Meeting another's goals, needs and desires will be a necessary requirement for satisfying one's own goals, needs and desires. The assumption is that while promoting the goals of others, one's own goals will be attended to by the person with whom one is interdependent (Markus & Kitayama, 1991, p. 229).

The concern for harmony over assertion of opinion means that in collectivist cultures there is often a preference for indirect and nuanced communication. Within collectivist cultures there is a greater reliance on the situation and on social context for understanding communication. As previously mentioned, in Vietnamese a term such as "uncle" carries with it meaning regarding the relative role and status of the person referred to, even when the "uncle" is not a relative. In contrast, in individualist cultures meaning is not very dependent on context (termed "low context communication"; Hofstede, 1991, p. 60).

In collectivist cultures members of the ingroup may be favoured over others in the allocation of desired objects or employment positions, for example. There are expectations that those who are in a position to allocate rewards will do so by favouring members of the ingroup (Hofstede, 1991). For example, bilingual-bicultural health professionals in Australia who provide services to persons of their own ethnicity are often expected to carry out "special favours" or make special efforts or allowances. They are considered by patients to be members of an ingroup defined by a common ethnic origin. Such health workers may want to help members of their ingroup; however, they are often trained in a Western model of clinical care, which takes as its basis an individualist relationship perspective for the clinician–client interaction. Within this framework requests for special efforts and favours would be seen as unjust and perhaps overly demanding. The lack of responsiveness from such health professionals often reflects the reality that they do not carry as much power in this society as their clients attribute to them. From the patient's point of view, however, the inability of the health professional to comply with requests may be seen as a lack of motivation to help on the part of the health worker and a transgression of very elementary obligations regarding interpersonal transactions. The health professional may be seen as disloyal to the patient and the ethnic ingroup and any therapeutic alliance may therefore be compromised.

If a special favour is done, particularly by a well-respected member of the community, an obligation is felt to repay the favour. This operates as a rule in most collectives, including those created within individualist cultures for the purposes of mutual benefit (e.g., reciprocal business referrals). When comparing cultures, those considered collectivist carry such arrangements into collectives like the family. Within ingroups there are mutual obligations of support. For example, many adult children from strongly collectivist cultures expect and are expected to repay a debt to their parents for having raised them. Such feelings and expectations in relation to the family may not be so prominent in a family that holds a more individualist attitude. Members of outgroups may also play an important role for ingroup members in collectivist cultures. When a member of the ingroup receives a favour from a member of the outgroup, particularly if the latter is perceived to carry status, then the obligation to return this favour is driven by the additional need to maintain face or the honour of the ingroup. Failure to meet obligations of reciprocation may invite alienation, conflict and shame.

Privacy and Involvement in the Group

In collectivist cultures there are fewer expectations of privacy from other members of the ingroup in relation to important decisions and actions. Private life is opened up to the group to allow family members to maintain an awareness of each other's needs in the interest of reciprocal interdependence and benefit (Markus & Kitayama, 1991; Shweder & Bourne, 1982). This raises questions about the cultural relativity of clinical terms such as enmeshment as given in the example at the beginning of this chapter. In collectivist cultures there are greater expectations by ingroup members that they will be involved with each other's everyday affairs than in individualist cultures. Age-related norms regarding privacy and involvement of the ingroup are different between individualist and collectivist cultures. For example, it would be normal for parents from a collectivist culture to want to monitor the courtship behaviour of their adult children, especially if they are female. There are often strong concerns about the moral integrity of a child's behaviour because the fallout from "immoral" activities can have widespread impact on the rest of the family (and, in many cases, the ancestral family). Mental illness in the family, in as far as it is stigmatised in a society, reflects on ingroup members more seriously in collectivist than in individualist cultures.

In individualist cultures where privacy of experience is emphasised, a transgression of cultural rules is typically associated with guilt. This is a private emotion that involves a person's inability to reconcile his own actions with reference to his own private moral standards. In collectivist cultures where emphasis is on social experience, shame rather than guilt is more typically experienced under similar circumstances. Here the experience reflects an inability to reconcile one's actions with reference to the collective's moral standards and transgressions represent breaches in the obligation of members of the ingroup to uphold the honour of the ingroup (Hofstede, 1991).

Understanding Behaviour: Individualist Versus Collectivist Perspectives

The cultural understandings of mental illness may be different depending on whether a culture is more strongly individualist or collectivist (see Box 2.3, Suicide and Culture — Durkheim's View). An interesting example of the differences in the understanding of suicide was given by a visiting Indian Ayurvedic[1] practitioner at the time when a major report was released that detailed youth suicide issues in Australia. He was puzzled and asked, "Why do young Australian people commit suicide?" The Australian mental health worker replied, "Maybe because they experience alienation and low self-esteem". The Indian practitioner said that this was strange to him; in India an unmarried woman who became pregnant might be expected to commit suicide (and may cause the suicide of her whole family) because of the shame brought upon the family name.

The relationship between individualism–collectivism and suicide was examined in a study by Minas, Read and Klimidis (1999). Individualism was found to be more strongly associated with male and female suicide rates across countries than collectivism. The authors cautioned against the broad assertion that values themselves could fully explain the suicide trends, stating that, "values emerge within a complex social, cultural, ecological and economic context". What they did suggest, however, was that:

> Individualism with its emphasis on uniqueness, the exercise of individual rights, responsibility to the self alone also cultivates isolation and alienation. Such a context may contribute to the propensity for suicide. Alternatively, sociocentric orientation and social integration with a cohesive ingroup, as in collectivist societies, may protect or prevent individuals from suicide (1999, p. 1).

Returning to the conversation between the Indian Ayurvedic practitioner and the Australian mental health worker, it is evident that two forms of explanation were given for suicide. In the case of the Australian mental health worker, internal personal attributes were given as reasons for suicide, while in the case of the Ayurvedic practitioner social and situational reasons were highlighted.

These differences in explanation relate to differences in the way that experience is structured in collectivist and in individualist cultures. In collectivist cultures actions are more likely to be seen as situationally determined and accounts of the actions will include the context, rather than inner dispositions. For example, Shweder and Bourne (1982) asked a cross-section of people in India and America to describe close acquaintances. Americans described people in terms of traits or personal characteristics. Rather than saying, "He does not disclose secrets", Americans were more likely to say, "He is discreet and principled". Americans were less likely to say, "He is reluctant to spend his money" than, "He is tight or selfish" (Markus & Kitayama, 1991, p. 232). Americans

---

1 Aruyveda is a wholistic system of medicine from India that provides guidance regarding food and lifestyle.

Box 2.3

Suicide and Culture — Durkheim's View

Research into suicide rates in individualist and collectivist cultures has a long history. Sociologist Emile Durkheim[2] (1897/1970) analysed differences in the rates of suicide in European countries during the mid-19th century, examining the contributions made by such factors as religion, marital status and age. In combination, the variations in suicide led Durkheim to conclude that "suicide varies inversely with the degree of integration of the social groups of which the individual forms a part" (p. 209). To illustrate, he contrasted the low rates of suicide of Catholics with the high rates of Protestants: both strictly prohibit suicide, but Protestantism "permits free enquiry to a far greater degree than" Catholicism (p. 157). "The Catholic accepts his faith ready made, without scrutiny ... A whole hierarchical system of authority is devised ... to render tradition invariable" (p. 158). If religion protects individuals against suicide, it is not because it preaches self-respect "but because it is a society" with strong collective states of mind embodied in shared beliefs, practices and traditions (p. 170). "When society is strongly integrated, it holds individuals under its control, considers them at its service, and thus forbids them to dispose wilfully of themselves" (p. 209). Accordingly, the evasion of societal duties through death is opposed. But when society's collective force weakens, individuals refuse to accept their subordination as legitimate and detach themselves from social life. An individual's personality will tend to prevail over the collective personality and he or she will depend only on his or herself and on rules of conduct that are based on self-interest. "If we agree to call this state egoism, in which the individual ego asserts itself to excess in the face of the social ego and at its expense, we may call egoistic the special type of suicide springing from excessive individualism ... So far as they are the admitted masters of their destinies, it is their privilege to end their lives. They ... have no reason to endure life's suffering patiently. For they cling to life more resolutely when belonging to a group they love, so as not to betray interests they put before their own" (p. 209–210).

Egoistic suicide is to be differentiated from altruistic suicide, which occurs in some cultures, not because the person "assumes the right to do so, but, on the contrary, *because it is his duty*. If he fails in this obligation, he is dishonoured and also punished, usually, by religious sanctions" (p. 219, emphasis in original). An example is the old Hindu custom that requires women to kill themselves when their husbands die. Suicide by an Indian girl and her family, because the girl is pregnant, may also be interpreted as altruistic. For society to be able to compel some of its

---

2   Émile Durkheim was a French social scientist who developed a vigorous methodology combing empirical research with sociological theory. He is widely regarded as the founder of the French school of sociology.

members to kill themselves they must belong to a highly integrated collective group, to the extent that the individual occupies "so little space in collective life he must be almost completely absorbed in the group ... [E]veryone leads the same life; everything is common to all, ideas, feelings, occupations" (p. 221). Whereas egoistic suicide "is due to excessive individuation", altruistic suicide is caused by insufficient individuation (p. 221). The individual "is only an inseparable part of the whole without personal value" (p. 221).

Durkheim further distinguished anomic suicide, which occurs as traditional societies give way to industrial expansion and economic prosperity. His analyses showed that suicide increased at times of industrial or financial crises, not because they caused poverty, but "because they are crises, that is, disturbances of the collective order ... Whenever serious readjustments take place in the social order, whether or not due to a sudden growth or to an unexpected catastrophe, men are more inclined to self-destruction" (p. 246). When society is disturbed in this way it is no longer able to exercise the moral restraint traditionally accepted as part of the collective order. The increased prosperity associated with industrial expansion leads to an increase in desires, but "when traditional rules have lost authority ... all regulation is lost for a time. The limits are unknown between the possible and impossible, the just and what is unjust ... Consequently, there is no restraint on aspirations" (p. 253). The more wealth individuals accumulate, the more dissatisfied they become because the horizons of their ambitions expand (Giddens, 1972). The race for an unattainable goal gives no satisfaction except for that of the race itself, but once the race "is interrupted the participants are left empty-handed. At the same time the struggle grows more violent and painful, both from being less controlled and because competition is greater ... Effort grows, just when it is becoming less productive" (p. 253). In this state of deregulation or anomy, Durkheim concludes that the desire to live is inevitably weakened and the likelihood of suicide increased. ■

also used situational descriptions, but this was more likely when they did not know someone well. In contrast, Indians described their friends in more situation-specific and relational terms than those used by the Americans. Indian respondents focused on the behaviour, on what was done, where it was done and to whom or with whom it was done.

Just as moral transgressions have wider effects on the ingroup in collectivist cultures, so too can positive qualities and achievements. In individualist cultures efficacy and expertise in task management or achievement are seen as strictly personal attributes. A doctor may carry no more worth than is carried by their expertise in delivering good medicine. In many collectivist cultures a doctor is invested with additional desirable attributes, abilities and powers to influence (this is discussed further below in relation to power distance). In collectivist cultures these qualities may also attach to those who share a familial association, friendship or acquaintance with such highly desirable persons. When a child achieves educationally the family also gains in status.

Power Distance

Power distance is the second value dimension that has important implications for the crosscultural clinical setting. This dimension is defined as "the extent to which the less powerful members of institutions and organisations (such as families, schools, the community and workplaces) ... expect and accept that power is distributed unequally" (Hofstede, 1991, p. 28). Power distance is the extent to which societies are structured hierarchically. In low power distance societies hierarchy is often viewed unfavourably. Holding power and exercising power over others is considered authoritarian and unjust. However, in high power distance societies, those in power and those less powerful collaborate in a mutually beneficial relationship. Attitudes towards the powerful are not unfavourable. Those in power are respected and obeyed, while those not in power can expect that the powerful will look after their interests and protect them. In low power distance societies the ideal is to minimise the differences between individuals in a hierarchy, whereas in high power distance societies the ideal is to maintain and observe differences in hierarchy.

In low power distance cultures egalitarian values are emphasised in interpersonal relationships. The focus is on minimising inequalities among people. Society emphasises equal rights and responsibilities. In high power distance cultures there is an acceptance that hierarchical relationships are natural and that life is structured by a wide series of dominant–subordinate relationships. As noted above, there is both an expectation that one holds a certain position within the society, and an acceptance of the roles afforded to this position. Those in authority are best described by the term of "benevolent autocrats", where the motivation for leadership is based on the view that they will govern according to the best interests of the populace. Those who are led entrust their leaders to make decisions for them and expect that these decisions will have their best interests in mind. Within high power distance cultures the concept of symbiosis is important between those who are leaders and those who are led. One cannot survive without the other. In contrast, those from low power distance cultures tend to view their leaders as accountable and their actions and motivations able to be questioned by the populace. Those who are led consider it their right to have a "say" in the decisions that are made about them, and share in the belief that a democratic process assures some control over the destiny of their lives. In workplaces subordinates may expect to be consulted rather than directed to carry out their work roles.

The basis for power distance can vary across societies, but can include status differences based on wealth, occupational position, age, gender, and role in the community. The currency used to define status differences varies across cultures. For example, in some Western societies privilege is given to youth, and young people are favoured with respect to both physical and psychological attributes. Most of the images aspired to, and driven by substantial advertising activity, involve young people who are agile and energetic, adventuresome, and free from responsibility. For those aged 40 years and over life is seen to be a decline into boorishness, weakness and frailty. The diminished value placed on older persons in some Western societies typically creates a significant pressure to remain youthful and to sustain roles that may indeed be quite unrealistic. In other cultures, where age is the basis of status, older members of the community participate in or have the responsibility for important decisions as well as providing many practical supports.

Across cultures there are significant variations in status based on gender, with females often seen, at least from a Western perspective, to carry subordinate roles. Indeed, value priorities are important to keep in mind when considering what may be labelled as "subordinate" or not. It is a value judgement to consider that women are subordinate to men if the criterion for dominance is based on the masculine role definitions defined in one society and applied to another. For example, some Western societies place a high value on independence, career-striving, risk-taking, and aggressiveness — all qualities typically attributed to the male gender role. From this perspective, nurturance and cooperation, which are qualities typically attributed to the female gender role, can be under-valued. Passing judgement on the roles of women from another culture, which may involve these latter attributes rather than the former, may be inaccurate, unfair and potentially offensive to these women. Actions taken during therapeutic contact based on these assumptions, such as encouraging women to assert their rights as defined by the counsellor in a family system, may lead to more harm than good to the women. This would amount to asking them to transgress the roles and expectations of their culture. While in some cases it might be appropriate to help with such transitions, therapists need to take into account how such transitions may be safely facilitated within the cultural context of this client. Similar comments apply to clinicians' prescriptions regarding adolescents' need to challenge the authority and power of their parents.

It is important to be aware that within any society there will be many currencies that define status differences and that these may differ between cultural groups. As noted, in many high power distance cultures those in positions of status, such as doctors or teachers, carry power. In such cultures, teachers may be seen as gurus who transfer personal wisdom, whereas in low power distance cultures teachers are more likely to be seen as experts whose role is to impart impersonal truths. In low power distance cultures subordinates expect to be consulted and to participate in decisions that are made, whereas in high power distance cultures subordinates expect to be told what to do. An outcome of the wide powers of influence given to authority figures within a high power distance culture is the emotional tone of relationships. Subordinates are expected to show respect towards their superiors. This sets the tone of many relationships, including employer–employee, teacher–student, parent–child, and doctor–patient.

In addition, there are differences between cultures in how power is acquired. In high power distance societies power is "inherited". In low power distance cultures there is greater mobility between status groups because greater value is placed on the personal possession of attributes that define status. The currency in low power distance cultures is such that it allows a greater mobility between groups because value is placed on attributes belonging to the individual. Individualist cultures, compared with collectivist cultures, provide greater opportunity for movement between different status groups. For example, the caste system that still exists in some parts of Indian society serves to rigidify the society so that its members are not able to move freely between the different social classes. This limitation applies both ways. Both those in power and those in more subordinate social positions are expected to strive for important social goals within their own status sphere. In individualist cultures socioeconomic upward mobility can be attained through intellect, which allows a person to obtain an education and enter in, or be identified with, a new group. In addition, in individualist cultures power currencies are often more fluid, with the potential for new currencies to be created and old currencies to become devalued compared with collectivist cultures.

Implications of Value Differences for Clinical Practice

Cultural values reveal the dynamics operating in interpersonal relationships, including those operating in the relationship between the client and clinician.

Let's return briefly to the clinical vignettes described early in this chapter. The clinician who described a Mediterranean client as a "mummy's boy" because he is still living at home at 30, made a value judgement based upon individualist values that people beyond a certain age should be independent from their families and self-reliant. The clinician was unaware that in a collectivist culture, which often may prevail in Mediterranean groups, there is an expectation that children will remain living at home until they marry. If they are sick, family loyalty dictates that the family will look after sick family members.

The clinicians who wondered why families were "such an issue in some cultures" also lacked awareness of these family values associated with collectivist societies. Furthermore, they may not have understood family distress at the privacy provisions that exist in mental health services, which interfere with the ability of the family to identify and respond to the needs of the sick family member.

The clinician who invited his Vietnamese client to address him by his first name spoke from the value position of a low power distance culture where it is expected that professionals and their clients will treat each other as equals. In many forms of Western psychotherapy, such as Gestalt therapy, equality between the clinician and the client is explicitly stated. But in a high power distance culture, such as in Vietnam, the client views and accepts the professional as superior and expects to treat the professional with respect and deference. The client would therefore feel disconcerted by the request to address the clinician by his first name. Similarly, the clinician showed a lack of understanding by assuming that he could address the client by his given name and may have potentially offended the client. It may be more respectful to ask by what name the client wishes to be addressed.

To further consider how value differences come into play in the clinical encounter we will use the following case study and other clinical vignettes to generate discussion.

A case example: Lin

Lin was born in a small province in China. She is the youngest of four children. As the youngest child in the family, Lin described herself as being loved and spoiled. She lived with her parents, two older brothers, their wives and children. Lin said that she was not required to do anything for herself because this was seen as the traditional role of her sisters-in-law. Lin said that she was a happy child, but very quiet and shy. Lin completed her high school studies and achieved well. She stated that she always had a couple of friends, and was very close to one of her sisters. She came to Australia at the age of 18 to live with her brother in the context of her parents becoming old and ill, and in order to pursue study opportunities. Her brother had been living in Australia since he first arrived as a refugee from the unrest associated with the Tiananmen Square massacre in Beijing in 1989.

Lin moved in with her brother and his wife (who was born in Australia but is of Chinese descent) and two young daughters. Her brother worked in a factory by day and a restaurant at night to support his family in Australia and back home. Her sister-in-law also worked long hours in a factory. Lin had no other relatives in Australia. Lin identified things as going wrong a couple of months after she started school. She expressed anxiety about travelling on public transport and said that she was stupid because she could not speak English properly. Lin also said that she felt that she was a burden on her brother and his family, that she was unable to properly care for her nieces and the house, and that her sister-in-law believed that she was lazy.

Lin was first referred to a community mental health clinic after some other students found her in the toilets, trying to cut her wrists. At that time she was assessed by the mental health crisis team and found to be experiencing both psychotic and depressive symptoms. She was hopeless, suicidal, believed that she was a ghost and a bad person and as a result of this was responsible for the problems of her family and the world. She said that she was "lazy and tired" and that she suffered from constant headaches. Lin was admitted, treated with antipsychotics and antidepressants and was discharged after two weeks. She was readmitted one week later and found to be non-compliant with her medication. This readmission was one of multiple admissions over a one-year period in which her medication and diagnosis changed a number of times. Some of the diagnoses she was given included bipolar affective disorder, schizoaffective disorder, major depression, dependent personality disorder and low IQ. Her family was described as unsupportive and family work was attempted but unsuccessful. The sister-in-law would not attend and only the brother spoke to staff. During the course of her treatment her fiancé broke up with her and Lin said that this was because he and his family thought she was "crazy".

Because Lin had difficulty continuing with her studies and was on a student visa, problems arose in regard to her ability to stay in Australia. The staff on the ward proposed that Lin return to China to be with her family. Lin was adamant that she could not return without a degree because if she did it would "kill her family". When this was also discussed with Lin's brother he said the same thing. The ward staff thought they were catastrophising and believed that Lin's family should accept her just for being her, regardless of her achievements.

Consider what cultural conflicts Lin may have encountered as part of her migration experience. She moved from a collectivist culture where she lived as part of a small community and was the youngest child in a tradition where she was not expected to carry much responsibility. It would have been the responsibility of her sisters-in-law in China to care for her. Her life in Australia involved a major role change: now she was an adult member of a small family unit with limited social supports and an aunt to young children, and therefore expected to contribute more. Lin was not much younger than her Australian-born sister-in-law, who needed her husband to support her and her children, so it is conceivable that another dependant in the family would create conflict. With Lin becoming unwell her need to be cared for would have increased and so would the stress upon the family. Lin was also required to travel to school independently on public transport, which would have been difficult to negotiate, given the cultural and language barriers, and given that independent travel would have been uncommon for Lin, even in China. Consideration of these psychosocial factors would be important in working with Lin, as would the cultural factors that impacted upon her diagnosis.

As already noted, Lin's diagnosis changed a number of times. The diagnostic uncertainty apparent in the change from a psychotic to a mood disorder raises some interesting questions about how culturally sanctioned behaviour can be differentiated from psychotic symptoms. (This is a topic that will be addressed in detail in chapters 5 and 6.) Issues relating to cultural values are raised by the Axis II diagnoses of low IQ and dependent personality disorder. Lin's IQ was not formally assessed and there are a number of problems in doing this across language and cultural barriers. As discussed in detail in chapter 4, a number of questions in intelligence tests are based on Western cultural values, items may have no cultural relevance, and translation of items may change or distort their meaning. In the absence of a formal assessment of Lin's intelligence and because Lin had limited English proficiency, judgements regarding her IQ may have seriously disadvantaged her.

A diagnosis of a personality disorder may also involve a value judgement as it is based on Western assumptions about normal development and, in the case of dependent personality disorder, on norms regarding dependence and independence that are specific to Western cultures. Lin's diagnosis of dependent personality disorder was based on her lack of independent living skills, both in the present and the past, and on her difficulty in adapting to the demands for independence placed on her by her new family and culture. It is true that Lin may have been unprepared for the migration experience; however, to diagnose her as being "dependent" is to pathologise the normative role of a youngest child in her culture. Contributing to the diagnosis of dependency may have been Lin's tendency to let her brother speak on her behalf and her lack of assertion within and outside her family unit. Once again, a cultural bias is evident — in collectivist cultures social harmony is valued over assertion and in high power distance cultures the less powerful or younger members of a family are expected to be dependent on the older or more powerful members.

The diagnosis of dependent personality disorder was also proposed by ward staff because of the observation that Lin's affect and behaviour were situationally unstable. For example, she was seen to be socially withdrawn from clinical staff yet animated with her peers and family. This observation reflects a further cultural bias. In an individualist culture, inner attributes or qualities, such as abilities, opinions and personality traits are understood to regulate behaviour and are, therefore, expected to be more or less invariant and constant over time and situation (Markus & Kitayama, 1991). In a collectivist culture, on the other hand, internal attributes are not understood to play a major role in regulating behaviour. A sense of an inner self may not be carried across situations, and behaviour may be determined by the demands of a situation. In explaining another's behaviour, members of interdependent cultures will refer to the context of the behaviour, rather than explaining it in terms of the individual's enduring traits or character. A stable and bounded sense of self underlies the theories of personality and personality disorder in Western psychiatry and psychology.

If the individual in a collectivist culture is understood to be one part of a whole, this has significant implications if he or she is separated from his or her social context. An example of this occurs when a person is admitted to hospital and the hospital has restrictive policies about visiting hours, discourages large groups of visitors, and will not permit family members to remain overnight with the inpatient. Provisions for privacy and confidentiality in mental health services restrict or even sever the opportunity for family members to identify and respond to the patient's needs. Separation from the family group during admission can cause great distress and confusion to patients from a collectivist culture.

The values of maintaining harmony and deference to hierarchy played a role within Lin's family unit and also operated in all of Lin's interpersonal relationships. These values are likely to have influenced Lin's ability to speak up in class, which is most likely to have been expected from her in an Australian educational setting. In Lin's previous educational experience she is more likely to have been directed as to what to do. In the clinical relationship there are similar expectations of clients. Lin may have been expected to speak up about the difficulties she had tolerating her medication, but this is likely to have been very difficult for her. Without an understanding of this, such behaviour becomes labelled as non-compliance. The lack of success in holding family meetings was related to the sister-in-law's unwillingness to attend and the brother's dominance. The Western family therapy model is based on a democratic family structure and on an openness in which family members are asked to share their private problems with strangers. These are not necessarily values held in collectivist, high power distance cultures.

A distinction may be made between the sharing expected from ingroup members and the privacy expected towards outgroup members. In clinical work it may be difficult for a clinician who is not part of the ingroup to elicit personal information from a patient who has been brought up in a collectivist culture. On the other hand, other difficulties may arise if the clinician is from the same collectivist culture. The client may perceive the clinician to have become part of their ingroup, once a relationship of trust has been established, and the client and family may develop expectations of a closer personal relationship and preferential treatment.

The importance to Lin of obtaining a degree, lest it "kill" her family, and the ward staff's lack of acceptance of this position, highlights the difference between cultures once again. For clinicians to argue that Lin should be accepted as an individual regardless of her achievements is valid in an individualist culture, but in a collectivist culture an individual's success or failure reflects on the whole family. This issue also highlights the importance of reciprocity. Lin was indebted to her family because of the great financial investment they had made in her future, the success of which was to belong to the whole family and the failure of which would shame the whole family.

Another case example that further illustrates the importance of reciprocity is provided by a Vietnamese woman who was in treatment at a community mental health clinic. She was experiencing serious financial difficulties and the stress of this was exacerbating her symptoms and impacting upon her recovery. Upon investigating the source of these difficulties the case manager discovered that this woman, who was married with three children, was not only supporting her immediate family but also sending money to her family in Vietnam. The case manager tried unsuccessfully to persuade the woman to focus on her family in Australia and stop sending money to Vietnam because she could not afford to continue doing so. She suggested that she be assertive with her family in Vietnam and that they would eventually understand that her income was not as great as it might seem from a Vietnamese perspective. This course of action seemed inconceivable to the client. The solution proposed by the case manager was based on an individualist value system that assumes that: the definition of the family is one of a nuclear family rather than the extended family; assertion to protect self-interest is more important than family harmony; and reciprocal obligations (her family helped her escape from Vietnam) could be forgone in favour of individual needs. This was in direct contrast to the collectivist value system held by the Vietnamese client.

In Summary

One of the main points we have made in this chapter is that clinicians need to consider whether cultural factors are important in the clinical relationship or in the case analysis. In doing this, clinicians should consider their own cultural position and what impact this may have on their interpretation of clinical information, and on the expectations that exist in the clinical relationship. Following are some useful questions for mental health workers to consider regarding how value systems may impact on the clinical relationship and on clinical information:

- Does the clinician come from an individualist or collectivist culture and from a high or a low power distance culture?

- Does the clinician's model of clinical practice derive from an individualist or collectivist culture or a high or low power distance culture?

- Does the client/family come from an individualist or collectivist culture or a high or low power distance culture?

- What are the bases of status in these cultures (age, gender, position) and do the client's and clinician's ideas of status agree?

- To what extent do the client, family and clinician adhere to the value orientations traditionally associated with their cultures, and what are the points of convergence or conflict between them?

- Are there important differences in value orientation between the client/family and the clinician and how do these impact on the clinical relationship?

- Are there important value differences between the client and the family members and how do these contribute to the client's difficulties?

- How do the client and the family perceive the clinician in terms of power?

- Is the clinician perceived to be a member of the ingroup or the outgroup and what impact does this have on the clinical relationship?

- With the progress of therapeutic contact are there changes to the status of the clinician in relation to the client/family?

Approaches to overcoming potential barriers created by value differences between client, family and clinician form part of the subject matter of chapter 7, Negotiating Explanatory Models.

Chapter 3

Expression and Communication of Distress Across Cultures

Key Points

▶ Clinical issues in the assessment of emotion

▶ Western assumptions about the expression of distress: depression and somatisation

▶ Understanding distress across cultures

The question of how well the diagnostic categories of Euro-American psychiatry fit the distress experiences of people across cultures was raised in chapter 1. Here we also examine this problem of "fit", but we emphasise the clinical issues that are raised in the assessment of emotion[1] across cultures. Difficulties in understanding the expression of emotions across cultures have been acknowledged in the clinical setting. In a survey conducted by the authors in 1998 of 180 Victorian mental health professionals, 55% acknowledged that their clinical skills were poorer when assessing mood and affect in clients of non-English-speaking background than in clients of English-speaking background (Stolk, 2002). Focus groups conducted with mental health clinicians also indicated they were uncertain whether they could accurately recognise emotions and emotional syndromes in their clients who were from a different culture to themselves. These clinicians agreed that they often experienced difficulty in determining whether a person of South East Asian background, for example, was showing signs of a depressive disorder. They had difficulties discerning whether a South East

---

1 The broad term emotion is used to discuss experiences such as sadness, anger and happiness. Emotion is defined as "a complex feeling state with psychic, somatic and behavioural components" that also incorporates the concepts of affect and mood (Kaplan, Sadock & Grebb, 1994, p. 300)

Asian patient's behaviour reflected a cultural tendency not to display emotion publicly or whether it reflected the presence of depression. Similar doubts were expressed in relation to people of a Mediterranean background. Clinicians said they were uncertain whether some Mediterranean clients were expressing emotion more "expansively" than Australians were typically accustomed to, or whether the clients' emotional expressions were symptoms of elevated mood associated with the manic episode of a bipolar disorder.

Clients of mental health services have also raised concerns about having their emotional expression misunderstood by mental health workers because of their cultural background:

> Eastern Europeans have a different temperament to [the] English. This is reflected in the way they show their emotions. Their interpretation of my excitability is as a manic condition. We talk louder, we move our hands more (Human Services, 1996, p. 19).

The conclusions that clinicians draw about the affective state of clients with a different cultural background to themselves influence the diagnosis reached and have important implications for the compliance with and the effectiveness of any treatments offered. Clients who feel they are not adequately understood or helped may not continue with the treatment and may also discourage others in their community from seeking available treatments and related services. There is a significant body of research reviewed by Klimidis, McKenzie, Lewis and Minas (2000) suggesting low participation by members of ethnic minority groups in mental health services provided in Western countries. The following case study illustrates the difficulty of trying to fit the distress experience of a non-Western client into a Western diagnostic system. The case also demonstrates the clinical implications this can have for an accurate understanding of the client's problem and for the effectiveness of treatment that might be offered in a Western mental health setting.

A Case Example: Thuy

This is a case study of a Chinese Vietnamese woman who attended an Australian mental health service after referral by a general practitioner (Cheung & Lin, 1997). The letter from the GP reads as follows:

> Dear Clinician,
>
> Thank you for seeing Mrs Thuy Nguyen, a 52-year-old Chinese-Vietnamese woman whom I have been treating for three months for complaints of fatigue, a range of muscle pains, sore neck and legs, accompanied by headaches. Investigations have failed to find evidence of a diagnosable physical disorder. As she has sometimes implied that she wishes she were dead, I am referring her to you for diagnostic psychiatric assessment.
>
> Yours faithfully
>
> Dr English

Presenting Symptoms

Thuy is a 52-year-old, Chinese-Vietnamese woman who complained of the following symptoms: extreme fatigue, difficulties with concentration, pains in her neck and legs, headaches, dizziness and difficulty sleeping. She said that at times she would become so distressed that she would wish she were dead. It was her thoughts about death that prompted her GP to refer her to a community mental health clinic for an assessment.

Current Circumstances

Thuy is a widow who lives with her elderly parents-in-law and her youngest son, who is in his final year of high school. Thuy has two older children who are married and living interstate. Thuy's parents-in-law are both elderly and frail and require constant care. As well as caring for them Thuy does shift work at a textile factory. Recently she had found it difficult to concentrate at work and the pain in her neck and legs has become quite debilitating. Thuy says that she is so tired that she is struggling to keep up with the overtime she is required to do. She said that because she has become slower at work her boss is expecting her to do overtime without being paid. Thuy said that she is too afraid to ask for more money for fear of losing her job. There has also been increasing pressure to do housework at home since her only daughter married and moved interstate 6 months ago. Her father-in-law constantly criticises Thuy for her failure to clean and maintain the house to its former standard. She worries constantly about money and is particularly concerned about not having enough to assist her son to pursue a tertiary education next year. He has suggested that he quit school to find work and Thuy feels guilty about this.

Personal History

Thuy, her husband, their two oldest children, and her husband's parents came to Australia as boat refugees in 1975. They worked very hard in a family restaurant which they were forced to sell 7 years ago when Thuy's husband became sick with cancer. He died 2 years after the business was sold and Thuy was left with debts to pay.

Past History of Symptoms and Treatment

Thuy first began to experience pain and fatigue 5 years ago, after her husband died. The pain has become increasingly debilitating over the past 6 months, however. For some time Thuy has consulted numerous GPs and specialists about her neck and leg pain and no treatment has been of help. She has been told that there is nothing physically wrong with her. Thuy describes her condition as one where life has become too much for her to bear and has worn her body down. She no longer believes that anything can help her.

In our training workshops the most common provisional diagnoses elicited by this case study from mental health practitioners were, in order: major depression, somatoform disorder, anxiety disorder and, less commonly, neurasthenia and chronic fatigue syndrome. In the following section these diagnoses will be discussed in terms of how well they provide an understanding of Thuy's complaints and what implications this has for treatment and clinical outcomes.

Depression, Anxiety and Somatoform Disorders

Depression, anxiety and somatoform disorders are all DSM-IV diagnoses that concern disturbances in mood and affect and carry several underlying assumptions about etiology and treatment. For the diagnosis of depression the following symptoms appear to fit Thuy's experience: fatigue, recurrent thoughts of death, loss of concentration, and disturbed sleep. The symptoms that cannot be readily accounted for by a diagnosis of depression are pain in her neck and legs, headaches and dizziness. An exclusion of these symptoms from the diagnosis is particularly problematic in Thuy's case, given that her physical symptoms were the primary complaint for which she first sought help. A diagnosis of an anxiety disorder could account for Thuy's complaints about fatigue and difficulties with concentration. Like the diagnosis of depression, however, it still provides an inadequate fit for the total sum of Thuy's complaints. The only DSM-IV diagnosis that takes into account Thuy's physical symptoms is somatisation disorder. Of all the DSM-IV diagnoses considered, this one gives primacy to the physical complaints that seem to cause her the most trouble. The diagnostic criteria require the presence of physical complaints that cause significant distress and impairment that cannot be explained by a general known medical condition. In the discussion that will follow in the section on somatisation, the apparent fit of this diagnosis to Thuy's complaint does not necessarily improve an understanding of her suffering, nor does it provide her with effective treatment options.

All of the possible DSM-IV diagnoses leave out something of Thuy's experience. Her symptoms cross over a number of different diagnostic categories. The omission of a significant part of Thuy's experience from the diagnosis has significant clinical implications for how effectively she will be understood and treated. The only diagnosis suggested that does not segment Thuy's experience and gives both primacy and validation of her physical complaints is neurasthenia. Neurasthenia is a diagnostic category in the ICD-10 and it is a major diagnosis in East-Asian countries (see Box 3.1 on neurasthenia). Neurasthenia is mentioned in the DSM-IV as the culture-bound syndrome *shenjing shuairuo*. The diagnosis of neurasthenia not only provides a better fit with Thuy's experience, but it also provides validation and an improved likelihood of effective treatment and resolution for Thuy. It can provide meaning to her condition that is shared by her culture of origin (see section on somatisation). Consider the opposite situation: a Western mental health worker visits a doctor in China complaining of lowered mood and lack of interest in normal activities — symptoms considered to be typical of depression. He is diagnosed instead with neurasthenia. The emphasis and primacy given to physical problems in this category of illness are likely to cause the mental health worker to think that the doctor has misunderstood his problem.

Box 3.1

Background on Neurasthenia

Neurasthenia includes symptoms of both major depressive and gener-alised anxiety disorders in which somatic symptoms are seen to be defin-ing rather than associated characteristics. It is a syndrome of exhaustion, weakness and various bodily complaints. Neurasthenia is believed to be caused by inadequate physical energy in the central nervous system (Kleinman, 1988). It is not seen as a mental disorder but rather as a popular and culturally sanctioned means of expressing distress.

Neurasthenia was first defined and popularised by George M. Beard in 1869, when he defined it as "a chronic functional disease of the nervous system" caused by the excessive expenditure of nervous energy. Beard was an American and saw the condition as being a peculiarly American phenomenon (Lin, 1989). Beard attributed the cause to sociopsychological stresses resulting from the rapidly advancing modern society, which had been uprooted from past traditions and values. Lin (1989) explains how this diagnosis was adopted by the East Asian cultures of China, Japan, Taiwan and Hong Kong. In the West, the concept of neurasthenia became outdated with the influence of psychoanalytic theory. This was because, according to Freud, anxiety occurred in the body (either as a feeling of anxiousness or somatic symptoms) by the repression of a thought (not a repression of affect). Problems of the body without a known biological cause came to be seen as connected to the mind (cognition). As early as 1894, Freud advocated the separation of neurasthenia from a particular syndrome called the anxiety neurosis. And henceforth, American psychiatrists diagnosed anxiety neurosis instead of neurasthenia.

Although neurasthenia lost favour in America, it remains important in the Chinese system of diagnosis. So much so that Lin (1989) describes neurasthenia as having been "transformed into a Chinese concept and indigenized in Chinese culture" (p. 117). Neurasthenia is a diagnosis that fits well in China because the distinction between the mind and body is not part of its historical and philosophical roots as it is in the West. According to Lin another reason for its continued popularity in East Asian cultures is because it serves to avoid the stigma associated with mental illness.

In a study by Kleinman (1980) of 100 patients in Hunan diagnosed with neurasthenia he reported that 87% could be reclassified as having

> depression. He treated this group with antidepressants and found that a number of them did not improve unless there was also some change in their social situation. These findings received a mixed response from Chinese psychiatrists. The term neurasthenia is used by half of the population of the world and to avoid ethnocentrism Lin proposed research that would look at whether patients in the US or Canada fit the diagnosis of neurasthenia — Kleinman's study in reverse. ■

As stated earlier, Thuy is most likely to receive a diagnosis in a Western mental health system of a disturbance of mood or affect — quite probably a diagnosis of depression. This diagnosis is based on a number of assumptions about the nature of emotion and the nature of the person that are particular to Western cultures and will be considered in the following section.

Western Assumptions about Emotion: Depression and Somatisation

> Western academically acquired knowledge cannot be separated from its cultural base even though it presents itself as our natural way of looking at the world (Lutz, 1985, p. 65).

When someone is described as depressed a culturally constructed judgement is made (Lutz, 1985) that carries many assumptions about consistencies in how people from different cultures think — not only about disorders, but also about things in general. Lutz (1985) argues that the "what and how of depressive experience and the dichotomy of 'emotion' and 'cognition' [may] make sense only in the context of the Euro-American cultural system within which they developed" (p. 63). While a construct such as "depression" may itself be a Western product, so too might the way we think about entities such as depression. One of Lutz's (1985) main points in this argument is that the *classification* of experience into fragmented and isolated constructs such as cognition and emotion may be strictly a Western product.

Different cultures have different configurations and classifications of experience and, therefore, understand, manifest and communicate distress differently. These differences are embedded within cultural knowledge systems that define what is knowable and how it is known, what constitutes reality (e.g., what forms of consciousness are admissible) and what constitutes deviance; for example, what is normal and abnormal (Lutz, 1985).

To understand the nature of this argument, the Western concept of depression, as an example, can be considered within a broader framework. The Western concept of depression is based on the following underlying assumptions:

• Depression is an internal personal phenomenon: Depression is assumed to be a problem that belongs inside the individual. In some cultures, however, similar emotions are framed as interpersonal or even situational. An intra-personal construction, on the other hand, seeks intrapersonal solutions, such as drug therapy or individual psychotherapy (Lutz, 1985).

• Depression is an abnormal state: Depression is assumed to be a disease or clinical entity that can be separated from the broader experience of human suffering and the pursuit of happiness.

• There are core biological emotions: It is assumed that all cultures experience and differentiate emotional experiences in the same way (e.g., depression and anxiety). Emotions are assumed to be primary experiences and are directly correlated to emotion concepts that are the same in all languages. This assumption is manifested in the way Western psychiatry views somatisation, a concept that requires a clear distinction between the mind and body (see section on Somatisation). The link between emotions and emotion concepts is further explored in the section Language and the Expression of Emotion.

The following sections will explore each of these assumptions futher.

Depression is Intrapersonal Not Interpersonal

An understanding of emotions as intrapsychic events, feelings or introspections of the individual is a specifically Western definition (Jenkins, Kleinman & Good, 1991, p. 70).

Historically the concept of depression placed greater emphasis on the social world in terms of its etiology, its meaning and its resolution. Nowadays depression is portrayed much more as a psychobiological phenomenon. Although current theory recognises that the onset of the disease might be triggered by social events in vulnerable individuals this is given secondary importance. In this context, cultural meanings associated with the experience are treated as distortions that need to be sorted out in an effort to get at the underlying biological cause (Good, Good, & Moradi, 1985).

Depression is seen as a disease of the mind. The domination of medicine in the conceptualisation of the mind attributes disorder to disease and the disease category is assumed to correspond to a natural physical phenomenon. When depression is viewed as a biological disease with different manifestations derived from culture and society then there is an exclusion of "the great cultural variation in the meaning of dysphoria, the great differences in cultural idioms for articulating distress, and the networks of meaning and experience" that ground the complaints (Good et al., 1985, p. 419).

In Western psychiatry, thought and emotion are considered the property of the individual located within the individual's mind. Emotion is conceptualised in psychiatry as a psychobiological fact and cognitive therapists propose that emotion is caused by thinking. Not all cultures conceive of emotions in this way. For example, studies of the Ifaluk in Micronesia suggest that for this group thoughts and emotions are not differentiated, nor are emotions internal to the individual. Rather, they are located between persons or within events or situations (Lutz, 1985). Across most cultures cognition and emotion are not separated from each other, or from action and the complex social world (Jenkins, Kleinman, & Good, 1991). Emotion in other cultures is thus rarely described as an autonomous internal experience.

Another way of approaching this issue is to consider the individualism–collectivism continuum introduced in chapter 2. The Western diagnostic system makes individualist assumptions about emotion. However, just as the self can be understood differently using the individualism and collectivism dimension so too can emotion. In some collectivist cultures emotions are defined within the interpersonal context rather than within the individual. This is illustrated in the attempt to translate the English concept "sad" into the Aboriginal language Pintupi (Wierzbicka, 1992). This example also highlights the problematic assumption that emotion concepts are universal, an issue that is expanded on later in this chapter.

Possible translations for the word "sad" into Pintupi include:

Watjilpa: preoccupation with thoughts of country and relatives. To become sick through worrying about them.

Wurrkulini: excessive concern for, and worry about, land or relatives, as for watjilpa.

Yiluruyiluru: dejection caused by worrying too much for absent relatives, for example, if they are in hospital.

Yirraru: as for watjilpa.

Yulatjarra: sympathy or sorrow for sick or deceased relatives. If a death has occurred this state is accompanied by self-inflicted wounds: "sorry cuts" (Wierzbicka, 1992, pp. 293–294).

What do these five possible translations from the English word "sad" into the Aboriginal language Pintupi suggest? The words "imply that the sufferer is 'worrying' for his land or his relatives" (Wierzbicka, 1992, p. 295).

In Micronesia, a person who experiences a prolonged period of mourning following the loss of a loved one is seen as not having found an adequate replacement for the lost relationship with another relationship (Lutz, 1985). In this case the problem (and its solution) is interpreted as taking place in the *interaction* between the person and the social and situational context. This has direct implications for psychiatric assessment, during which the process of reaching a diagnosis depends partly on eliciting individualistically oriented self-statements. The question, "What are you really feeling?" is based on the assumption that ultimate social reality is internal. Such an assessment runs the risk of failing to elicit adequate information from the client and can lead to a negative value judgement being made by the clinician. This is because in Western cultures, and particularly in psychiatry and psychology, introspection is highly valued. Introspection, however, plays a different role in different societies; in some societies social insight is more highly valued than individual insight. Some cultures view feelings as private and embarrassing events that should not be explored, as they are generally not perceived as the cause of distress (Kleinman, 1986; Lutz, 1985).

In his interviews and psychotherapy with Taiwanese students, Kleinman (1980) found it extremely difficult to elicit personal ideas and feelings even after a trusting relationship was established. He found that the orientation of most of the Taiwanese was outward rather than inward, and unlike many middle-class Caucasian Americans they had very little past experience of self-scrutiny to draw upon. He reported two types of feelings: those that were — from a contemporary Western perspective — superficial and unreflective, and those feelings that were held to be deep or private that were never shared with anyone, except on special occasions with intimate friends. Many informants asserted that these deeply held ideas and feelings were the only privacy they possessed and to ask about or freely talk about such matters was embarrassing and shameful. The cultural norms governing interpersonal transactions protect one from ever having to communicate one's most private inner world.

Bhurga and Bhui (1997) suggest that the preoccupation with psychological insight in Western cultures might be viewed as self-absorption in other cultures. A good example of the way that introspection is viewed is found in a form of Japanese psychotherapy, called Morita therapy, which discourages patients from talking about their problems and from complaining about their symptoms and encourages them instead to think of others (Tseng, 1999).

Depression is an Abnormal State

In Western society, affects pertaining to sorrow are "free floating" that is, they are not linked to an ideology but rather are observable in isolation and conducive to being labelled as illness.

Obeyesekere (1985) states:

> ... this need not be the case in other societies where these affects do not exist free-floating but instead are intrinsically locked into larger cultural and philosophical issues of existence and problems of meaning (p. 135).

Studies of depression across cultures can be criticised as an example of a category fallacy in that symptoms are isolated from their cultural context (see chapter 1). "While it is true that the disarticulation of symptoms from context will facilitate measurement it is also likely that the entities being measured are empty of meaning" (Obeyesekere, 1985, p. 137).

In many non-Western cultures depression is not an illness or a negative state that needs to be avoided and treated (Obeyeskere, 1985; Swartz, 1998). In Buddhism sadness and sorrow are seen as part of the nature of life itself and "[t]he ordinary person knows that the world is perforce one of suffering" and sorrow (Obeyeskere, 1985, p. 139). Therefore, an individual's expression of feelings of hopelessness is not a symptom of depression but of life itself. According to Buddhism, the cause of suffering is desire or craving, and by following a path of learning, which involves renunciation of desire, insight can be gained. Both sadness and sorrow in life belong to the realms of the world of pleasure and domesticity that are illusory and transitory. The path entails meditation and renunciation of attachments, both physical and emotional. Past deeds in earlier incarnations are believed to affect a person's contemporary life, and insight into this can release the individual from the burden of future incarnations and open the way towards enlightenment. In this instance there is a risk of misconstruing a spiritual quest as symptoms of depressive illness. An example of this happened to Obeyeskere (1985) when a visiting American colleague commented to him that one of his friends was depressed. Obeyeskere responded that his friend was not depressed, he was a Buddhist.

Another example of a culture in which depression has a different value and meaning is in Iran. In Iranian culture suffering and grief are perceived as enobling and socially valued. For example, a sad person with a tragic life is regarded as being someone with a depth of inner self; while a happy person may be regarded as being shallow and socially incompetent (Good et al., 1985). In Iranian society dysphoria is "religiously motivated grief, an experience of personal depth, and a positively valued perspective on the tragic character of the social order" (Good et al., 1985, p. 420).

There are Core Biological Emotions
Differentiation of Emotion States

In Western cultures it is traditional to develop:

> Understanding of things by breaking them into smaller and smaller parts; and the model of the machine made up of smaller and smaller components has been used to develop understandings not only of mechanical things, but also of people (Swartz, 1998, p. 105).

In Western psychiatry and psychology it is assumed that emotions can be clearly separated into distinct categories. The differentiation of emotion states is highly valued because it is necessary for diagnosis of, for example, anxiety disorders or major depression. Diagnoses, in turn, direct the clinician to loosely corresponding treatment options. Regardless of the person's "actual" experience, the DSM-IV treats symptoms such as anxiety and depression as belonging to separate categories. The diagnosis of neurasthenia is an example of an alternative way of conceptualising symptoms of distress, in which anxiety, depression and somatic symptoms are not separated from each other (Lewis-Fernandez & Kleinman, 1995). Interestingly, research suggests that these symptoms generally are not experienced as separate by patients.

Leff (1988) found that patients were less likely to differentiate depression from anxiety than psychiatrists expected they would be. He suggested that psychiatrists are harbouring "idealised disease concepts, despite the fact that patients usually exhibit a mixture of the symptoms" (Leff, 1988, p. 71). The problem with this research is the conclusion that Leff drew, which was not that psychiatrists do not fully understand the clients' experience, but rather that psychiatrists are at the leading edge in terms of understanding emotion.

According to Swartz (1998), this theory implies that being able to differentiate emotions is of greater value than not having this ability, and that the more differentiated emotions are for the individual the better the implications for treatment. As Swartz (1998) argues, there is no reason to assume that experiencing one's emotions in a way that is more familiar to psychiatrists is any better or more sophisticated than any other way. Furthermore, belonging to a culture that does not differentiate emotions the way Western psychiatry does may disadvantage people from other cultures if they are seeking Western mental health services.

Somatisation

The concept of somatisation or psychosomatic illness has arisen as a relatively recent phenomenon in Western thinking, and is derived from the distinction made between the mind and the body, which non-Western cultures tend not to make (Lutz, 1985).

According to Stekel, somatisation is:

> A type of bodily disorder arising from a deep-seated neurotic cause. It is as if the organs of the body were translating into a physiopathological language the mental troubles of the individual (as cited in Campbell, 1996, p. 677).

Along the same lines, Campbell (1996) defines somatisation as "the organic expression of mental processes" (p. 677).

Somatisation has been defined according to a number of accounts of its mechanisms. These include:

- As a psychological mechanism in which there is an externalised cognitive response to stress.

- In some psychodynamic views as an immature defence.

- In anthropological and cultural psychiatry as a coping mechanism.

- As serving a social function and as being due to the lack of words or concepts to describe feelings of sadness.

All of these theories suggest that "the unexpressed emotion is metamorphosed into a physical symptom" (Escobar, 1987, p. 175). As we discuss below, the diagnosis of somatisation raises several problems crossculturally. The general problem with the Western model is that it can invalidate other ways of experiencing and describing distress by trying to fit the individual's expression into the Western professional categories. Furthermore, symptoms may not be explored in any detail because there is no corresponding treatment option.

The Superiority of Psychological over Somatic Symptoms

The definitions of somatisation imply that emotional distress is transformed into bodily experience. In fact, there is no conclusive empirical support for this assertion. Therefore, it is no more empirically valid (or invalid) than asserting that "spirit possession" is responsible for emotional distress. Phan and Silove (1997) report that "there is no conclusive empirical evidence for the widespread assumption that somatic symptoms are substituted for affective symptoms in Vietnamese culture" (p. 87). Others agree. According to research by Robbins and Kirmayer (1991), "the assumption that somatisers have an underlying major psychiatric disorder that accounts for their physical distress is more often wrong than right" (p. 134).

Since the beginnings of cultural psychiatry the concept of somatisation has been associated with Chinese psychopathology (Cheung, 1995). Some of the reasons suggested to explain why Chinese people somatise include: denial, suppression or repression of emotions, failure to differentiate between the mind and the body, or social suppression of psychological symptoms, with the consequence that distress must be expressed physically (Cheung, 1995).

There is a clear ethnocentric bias in this perspective. As Lewis-Fernandez and Kleinman (1995) assert, the majority of humanity displays a more somatic than psychological expression of distress. Nevertheless, Western clinicians treat physical symptoms as a special category because patients are expected to adopt "an exclusively psychological idiom for their distress" (Kirmayer, 1996, p. 152).

Whereas the Chinese have been "accused" of "somatising", Western cultures could equally be accused of "psychologising" their distress (Sue & Zane, 1987). If somatisation is viewed as a defence mechanism then it is implied that a psychological way of seeing the world is given privilege. Accordingly, the psychological process is given primacy over the physical expression. In adopting this position, however, there is a loss of the meaning that somatic expressions of distress may communicate within a particular culture. Furthermore, if the psychological expression of distress is seen to be primary then there is the danger of falling into the same trap as evolutionist theorists such as Leff (1973), who rank the physical manifestation of distress as somehow inferior or less "sophisticated" than its emotional manifestation.

Somatisation, Validation and Stigma

Whereas diagnoses of physical disorders such as neurasthenia may serve to avoid the stigma of mental illness in China and other Asian countries, the diagnosis of somatisation disorder in the Western biomedical system does not. There is stigma associated with pain when such pain is believed to have no biological cause. If a condition is not seen to be "real" (as in having a physical origin) then there is a danger that the associated pain may not be seen as real either. The outcome of this position is to invalidate the experience of the patient. In our training sessions, clinicians who diagnosed Thuy as having chronic fatigue syndrome also joked that this was a "Mickey Mouse diagnosis". Those diagnosed with chronic fatigue syndrome, fibromyalgia and irritable bowel syndrome report a great deal of suffering associated with not being seen to have a valid diagnosis (Kirmayer & Robbins, 1991).

Several authors report that patients who present with somatic symptoms feel profoundly misunderstood when offered a psychiatric explanation for their distress. Even if the patient does present with dysphoria, this is more likely to be understood by the patient as a consequence rather than as a cause of the physical distress (Robbins & Kirmayer, 1991). According to Ragurum, Weiss, Channabasavanna and Devins (1996):

> The social meaning of somatic symptoms is less distressing because they closely approximate experiences that everyone has from time to time. Depressive symptoms on the other hand are considered to be private and even dangerous (p. 1048).

The situation applies in reverse in many Western clinical settings where psychotherapy is in favour. Here psychological symptoms are more likely to be reported than somatic symptoms as a result of the relative social desirability of such symptoms (Raguram et al., 1996). In addition, demand characteristics of Western clinical settings communicate to patients who can understand the language of such settings that they are expected to report psychological symptoms. Patients from other cultures who often do not understand this "language" fail to respond to the expectations of such settings. In such settings, stripped of the cultural context, their "natural" expression of distress is interpreted as alien, it is mislabelled and can potentially be regarded as invalid.

A diagnosis that is culturally "sanctioned" within Asian communities, such as neurasthenia, provides a meaningful framework for understanding the experience of the sufferer and for responding to it. It can provide validation of Thuy's (our earlier case study) experience for her family and for the broader cultural community of which she is a member. The diagnosis also provides possibilities that can be drawn upon from within the social network for its resolution. For example, any changes in her roles and interactions with others and the environment are more likely to be seen as legitimate measures in response to her illness.

Thuy was experiencing multiple social demands from work, where she was required to work overtime by her boss, and from home, where she was required to manage the household and care for her ageing in-laws and son. These events occurred in the background of numerous stresses, including the death of her husband, financial pressures and the departure of her daughter from home. Thuy felt culturally bound to maintain her roles, which were becoming increasingly difficult for her to manage. Sicknesses aside, there were no culturally sanctioned options for her to draw upon for the resolution of her social and situational difficulties. According to Kleinman (1986) and others (Littlewood & Lipsedge, 1987), somatic symptoms can be a form of protest or exaggeration of disorder by those who occupy an inequitable position within the social order. Somatic symptoms may be a way of engaging in the world and may serve to communicate social and situational difficulties. Kleinman (1988) suggested that somatisation ought to be considered as a way of experiencing and expressing distress without words. If Thuy's distress is considered outside the parameters of Western psychology and psychiatry her distress does not need to be interpreted as a transformation of an internal conflict into a physical expression. It can instead be understood as an expression of her social and situational difficulties, not as secondary to some more "important" psychological process. There is clearly a problem in separating a person's experience of illness from its cultural and social context. The Western diagnostic system removes the individual from the social context by diagnosing the disorder as intrapersonal rather than interpersonal and situational.

Language and the Expression of Emotion

Having "the" Vocabulary

An obvious set of difficulties in assessing and understanding emotion across cultures stems from the lack of language equivalence and the dynamic nature of languages. In crosscultural clinical work mental health workers are surprised to learn that the client's language "lacks" particular emotion terms (e.g., Vietnamese has no direct translation for the word "depression"). It must be recognised, however, that languages differ in the availability of specific terms to label emotional experience. Chinese, for instance, has a rich vocabulary of 750 terms for emotions compared to English, which has 400 words (Heelas, 1996). The absence of a direct translation of an English term does not mean that a language lacks words or broader statements (e.g., common metaphors) to describe similar emotion states. Furthermore, the absence of an equivalent word to describe an emotion does not mean that as a *construct* that emotion is lacking in that language group. Stating that another language or culture "lacks words" is a relative judgement based on the assumption that English is the standard language. At the same time, such a statement may reflect the difficulties and frustrations mental health workers experience as they attempt to communicate with someone from another culture on their own terms. This attempt is likely to be further hampered by the fact that our thought processes are structured by our culture and language, which may not be how other cultures structure their thinking. Communication barriers may exist even within the English language. English, as a natural language, will often differ in different regions of the world or within sub-cultural groups living in the same region. For example, the term "user-friendly" has crept in to the English language among professionals who are exposed to computers, but this term is meaningless to others who "speak" English but are not members of this sub-culture.

Language and Metaphors of the Body

Metaphorical and contextual expressions of psychological symptoms may be misinterpreted as being somatic symptoms. For example, a "broken heart" and "butterflies in the stomach" are metaphors particular to English. Other metaphors exist in other cultures and languages; for example, "swallowing frogs" denotes anger in Brazil (Becker, 1994). Metaphors are obviously embedded within semantic structures shared by a cultural group. The understanding of metaphorical terms requires interpretation from within that culture.

English Emotion Concepts Are Not Universal

We have already suggested that the concept of emotions as biological or factual can be seen as a Western, ethnocentric perspective. From this angle, then, emotions cannot be assumed to be the same across cultures. Culturally different interpretations of the self and of emotion suggest qualitative differences in the experience itself (Jenkins et al., 1991). Experience cannot be separated from its sociocultural and linguistic context. This is because the primary language used to describe the experience is the same language that first differentiated and gave a name to this experience. It can be argued that distress and suffering are universal, but the concepts, their meaning and their manifestations are culturally and linguistically determined.

Interpersonal communication that shares the same language and the same sociocultural conditions facilitates the expression of experience. When the experience is communicated across linguistic and cultural boundaries there is a loss of information, meaning and understanding. There is a problem in assuming that the experience of the sickness and the expression of the symptoms can be clearly and unambiguously separated (Herzfeld, 1986). This is because another's experience is judged from their behaviour and speech and cannot be accessed without the filter of language and culture. A major aspect of the study of emotion across cultures involves the study of language.

According to Kirmayer (1992) psychiatry tends to treat language more as a universal code (a literal statement about an object) rather than as a personal expression. Words such as happiness, sadness, anger, fear and anxiety are not core universal emotion concepts — rather they encode concepts specific to the English language. Wierzbicka (1992, p. 287) states that "there are no emotion terms that can be matched neatly across language and cultural boundaries". One example of this was provided earlier in this chapter in the attempt to translate the English concept "sad" into Pintupi. The translations suggested that these words were "not really words for sadness, depression or worry" but "words for something else" (Wierzbicka, 1992, p. 295).

It is not the case, therefore, that all languages in the world have words that correspond to what the English language identifies as "basic emotion concepts" such as happiness and anger. To assume that these *are* basic emotion concepts is an ethnocentric perspective. This does not mean that there are no emotions that are universal. It means that emotions cannot be matched across languages, given that words are more than just words — they embody language-specific and culture-specific concepts. There is a difference between saying there are no universal emotions and there are no universal *emotion concepts*.

Emotion concepts are specific to a language and culture, and people inherit and learn concepts such as "anger" and "sadness" from their culture to distinguish types of events. People from different cultures also differ in terms of what they feel emotion about. For example, being told what to do elicits anger in some and deference or respect in others (Shweder, 1985). English emotion concepts, therefore, do not have a privileged status.

There are differences in the socialisation of affect that are rooted in the social development of persons within a culture. "The tendency to perceive and report distress in psychological or somatic terms is influenced by various social and cultural factors" (Ragurum et al., 1996, p. 1043). Different cultures emphasise different emotions, because these emotions have different cultural values and meanings. For example, Iranians and Mediterraneans encourage displays of sadness and sorrow, whereas Anglo-Celtic cultures tend to foster stoic endurance. The Chinese discourage excessive expression of emotion because it is seen to disrupt social harmony and cause sickness. For the Ilongot anger is believed to be so dangerous that it can destroy society, while the Inuit view anger as a child's experience. Similarly the Tahitians do not value, and therefore rarely express, anger. For the Americans anger is more highly valued because it is believed that it can help overcome fear and lead to independence (Shweder, 1985).

A Culturally Sensitive Approach to Understanding Emotion and Distress

So far we have discussed some of the problems that may be encountered in assessing emotion across cultures, and the implications for how well understood and helped an individual from a non-Western culture might feel in a Western mental health setting. We consider now how some of the barriers to understanding can be overcome through the development of a culturally sensitive approach. First and foremost, a culturally sensitive approach requires an awareness of the ethnocentric biases inherent in the mental health worker's model of understanding. It is here that the barriers need to be identified rather than being attributed to the client or their culture. A culturally sensitive approach requires sensitivity to the social context, and the client's personal and social history. An emic approach that is characteristic of ethnographic studies (see chapter 1) may provide a model that will yield a greater understanding of the client than will an attempt to fit cultural variations into an ill-fitting nosological framework (Kirmayer, 1996).

The aim of an emic approach is to understand the personal meaning of the illness and suffering for the individual, their family and their community. To this end, Swartz (1998) recommends a "meaning centred approach", which recognises "the diversity of emotional experience in different contexts" (p. 108). Swartz states:

> When we are told, then, for example, that guilt may be less of a feature of depression in non-Western cultures than in the West, or that sadness may be replaced by bodily complaints, our task is not to look for the ways in which some people may not fulfil standard biomedical criteria of what constitutes depression. It is rather to attempt to understand what the particular pattern of symptoms means in the context within which the person lives (p. 109).

In the process of seeking a greater understanding, a clinician can ask a number of questions: of themselves, of the client and family, and of other people in the client's community (see Box 3.2, Facilitating Assessment of Emotion Across Cultures). For example, "To what extent does the meaning system of the client correspond to your own?"

For Thuy a culturally sensitive approach suggests that an understanding of her suffering should be sought in the context in which she lives. A clinician might ask, "What does it mean to be a widowed Chinese-Vietnamese woman living with her in-laws?" and "What meaning does Thuy give to her suffering in terms of her cultural beliefs?"

Thinking about suffering and pain in a more empathic and creative way requires stepping outside assumed categories and interpretations. An awareness of the following issues underpins a culturally sensitive approach:

- The clinician is the instrument by which the client's verbal and non-verbal behaviours are interpreted.

- Clinical interpretations are determined both by the clinician's values and by the values that underpin the diagnostic system used.

- Each idiom of distress is part of a meaning system (it is never enough to describe someone as "just somatising").

- The meaning of a particular pattern of symptoms may be found in the context within which the person lives (Swartz, 1998).

- A culturally sensitive approach recognises the client as the expert in their own suffering.

- The client's understanding of the body, the mind, and illness is likely to be different to that of the clinician. This requires the clinician to work within the client's framework as much as possible.

- Negotiation occurs within the shared space between clinician and client.

Box 3.2

Facilitating Assessment of Emotions Across Cultures

In consultation with a group of 11 bilingual case managers the authors developed the following principles to facilitate assessment of emotion across cultures, some of which reiterate and summarise points we have made earlier:

• Establish a relationship; listen to the client's story and allow the meaning of the story to emerge. Allow clients space to express distress in their idiom.

• Recognise the expectations the client may have of you (e.g., regarding your expertise).

• Ask permission to ask questions. Don't be intrusive. Take time.

• Explain to the client and family why you're asking questions as the questions might seem strange to them.

• The client and family may be accustomed to an indirect approach in interviewing and it may be respectful to employ this rather than asking questions directly.

• Listen to what the family interpret as normal or abnormal. This may aid in identifying the social issues that may be contributing to the client's distress.

• Assess comprehensively by remembering to take the social and cultural context and meaning into account. ■

In the final chapter we explore the process of negotiating a shared understanding between the client and clinician in greater detail. In the following chapter we will elaborate on some of the practical issues involved in translating emotion terms and psychological tests and measures.

Chapter 4

Issues in Translating Mental Health Terms Across Cultures

Key Points

▶ Language connotations

▶ Working with interpreters

▶ Cultural relevance of tests and measures

Translating Emotion Terms

> People who speak different languages live in different worlds; not in the same world with different labels attached. (Sapir, 1980, as cited in Marcos, Urcuyo, Kesselman & Alpert, 1973b, p. 658).

In this chapter we examine problems that can arise when mental health terminology is translated from one language into another, whether in a clinical interview or in a psychological assessment instrument.

The goal of translation is to communicate the same meaning in the second language that was communicated in the first (Larson, 1984; Westermeyer & Janca, 1997; Bontempo, 1993). Words that describe emotions tend to be abstract and language specific, which means they are not easily translated. For example, the word "depression" in English can be translated in five different ways into Vietnamese. One of these Vietnamese terms for depression carries strong connotations of anxiety. If the patient agrees that they are having this experience, they may be misunderstood by a Western clinician as having agreed that they are depressed (Phan & Silove, 1997). When a term is translated literally, it may acquire new and unintended connotations, so that its meaning is not actually equivalent to the term in English (Westermeyer & Janca, 1997). Consequently a different meaning structure is being elicited.

Unintended Connotations

Unintended connotations were elicited when the World Health Organization attempted to translate the Self Reporting Questionnaire (SRQ), a measure that assesses a range of symptoms including the depression syndrome. When the mental health terms in the SRQ were translated and administered in Amharic (an Ethiopian language) Kortmann (1987) found that responses reflected a different meaning structure than the instrument was designed to measure. A literal translation of "Do you feel unhappy?" received the common response "No, because no-one has died". The concept "unhappy" appears not to exist as a separable phenomenon in this culture but instead it is strongly associated with a clear cause or situational context. The question, "Do you cry more than usual?" was interpreted as asking whether the person had attended more funerals than usual. The question, "Is your appetite poor?" was interpreted as a question about the availability of food. The question, "Do you sleep badly?" was interpreted as a question about nightmares or sleep-walking (Kortmann, 1987).

Intended Connotations Are Difficult to Convey in Translation

Emotion terms in each language have specific connotations and associations that often cannot be accurately translated by a corresponding word in another language (Phan & Silove, 1997). The specific cultural connotations of health terms may be lost when translated into English from a language other than English. The meaning of health terms may depend on a traditional medical model (e.g., Chinese medicine). Or terminology may be based on, for example, Confucian or Buddhist principles, meaningful only to followers of those beliefs.

Words may have metaphorical meanings, which may be lost in translation, as for example in the English "butterflies in the stomach" or "a broken heart". The term "heart distress" in Iran has metaphorical connotations and does not refer to angina or an impending heart attack (Good & Good, 1982).

Translation into Vietnamese of the item "feeling low in energy, slowed down" in the Hopkins Symptom Checklist emphasises physical weakness or lethargy, but "does not convey adequately affective tone intended by the item" (Phan & Silove, 1997, p. 88).

Lay Terms Should Be Avoided

Lay terminology and jargon can be very difficult to translate accurately and should be avoided. For example, the English word "blue", sometimes used as a lay term for depression, in Vietnamese means "hope" or a state of "calmness". In Russian slang, "blue" means drunk, while in German "blue" can be used to refer to someone who is gay.

Working with Interpreters Requires Skill

The foregoing issues in the translation and interpreting of mental health terms illustrate that mental health interpreting is a *professional* skill (Ebden, Bhatt, Carey & Harrison, 1988; Marcos, 1979). Marcos (1979) and Ebden et al. (1988) recorded psychiatric interviews using lay interpreters, such as other patients, friends, relatives or non-accredited hospital staff. They found that these interpreters introduced a range of distortions due to lack of language competence, lack of psychiatric knowledge, and the interpreter's attitude. Ebden et al (1988) found that out of 143 questions and answers, more than 80 terms were mistranslated, misunderstood or not translated. The more complex the question, the greater the number of mistranslations. It should be clear, therefore, why family members (particularly children) or other lay people should not be used to act as interpreters (Marcos, 1979) (see Box 4.1, Working with an Interpreter). To ensure that an accurate translation is made of the client's and the clinician's communications it is important to work collaboratively with the interpreter.

Cultural Elaboration Is Often Necessary

Even if words such as "depression" or "anxiety" cannot be translated exactly into a language other than English, it is still possible to elicit from the client their experience of distress. "This may require several sentences in language A to describe the feeling in a single word of language B" (Westermeyer & Janca, 1997, p. 297). This process may be described as the "cultural elaboration of emotional experiences" (Westermeyer & Janca, 1997, p. 297). Many clinicians have observed that the interpreter sometimes appears to speak for longer than their client or themselves; the need to elaborate a particular term may be one of the reasons for this.

Choosing a Language for Assessment

Research has shown that the language in which a bilingual client is assessed can affect ratings of level of psychopathology. For example, Marcos et al. (1973) found that native Spanish-speaking patients, who also spoke English and who were diagnosed with schizophrenia, were rated by psychiatrists as having a higher level of pathology when interviewed in English than in Spanish, even when they appeared competent in English. In English, the patients spoke slowly, hesitated and paused frequently, showing signs associated with depressed mood or defensiveness, and so they were diagnosed with a greater level of pathology than when they were interviewed in Spanish (Marcos, Alpert, Urcuyo & Kesselman, 1973; Marcos, Urcuyo, Kesselman & Alpert, 1973).

When assessing a client who is bilingual it is important not to overestimate the client's English proficiency, because emotion and mental health terms are much harder to express in a second language than in a first. Although clients might be able to conduct an everyday conversation in English, they may not be sufficiently proficient in English to discuss their psychological state or to understand and participate in a clinical discussion of diagnosis and treatment (Stolk, 1996; Westermeyer & Janca, 1997). The client's current level of psychopathology may also affect their level of English proficiency (Oquendo, 1996). Patients who are well may speak English fluently, but during a psychotic episode may, for a time, revert to their first language and be unable to communicate in English (Stolk, 1996).

The client should be asked in which language they are most fluent and would prefer to be assessed. The clinician, however, also needs to exercise judgement and decide whether the client is currently sufficiently proficient in English to discuss clinical matters in English. If there are doubts about the client's English proficiency, then an interpreter should be engaged or the assessment should be conducted by a bilingual clinician (Del Castillo, 1970; Marcos, Alpert et al., 1973; Marcos, Urcuyo et al., 1973; Marcos & Alpert, 1976; Oquendo, 1996, Ziguras et al., 2000). A bilingual assessment allows the client to switch languages if they wish. In this way information may be obtained that may be overlooked due to language independence (Oquendo, 1996). This is a phenomenon in which some affective experiences may become separated from the content to which they are related because these experiences are accessible in one language but not in the other (Marcos, 1976; Marcos & Alpert, 1976; Oquendo, 1996). People who are bilingual may have duplicate stores of meaning, each of which may be accessible only by its respective language (Marcos, Urcuyo et al., 1973). Psychological experiences such as depression or anxiety may be "bound" to the language spoken (Marcos, Urcuyo et al., 1973, p. 658).

The Three-way Dynamic

Communicating through interpreters raises issues that occur as a result of the very presence of the interpreter. The presence of this third person inevitably changes the nature and structure of the interaction between client and clinician.

A study by Kline, Acosta, Austin and Johnson (1980) examined how patients and doctors in a mental health outpatient setting responded to the presence of interpreters in initial interviews. Patients interviewed with interpreters said that they were generally better satisfied with the clinic service, felt more helped by the doctors, and felt more understood than those interviewed without interpreters. It was found that the doctors tended to actually underestimate the degree to which clients seen with interpreters felt helped. They also indicated that they were not comfortable about seeing this client group beyond the initial interview. The authors suggest that the lack of precision between speech, body movement and facial expressions can make the therapist unsure and uncomfortable. Also, when working through an interpreter it takes twice as long as an uninterpreted interview to gather and convey information. The interruption to the flow of speech and thought that is an inevitable part of an interpreted interview can interfere with effective communication when complex or emotional information is being imparted. For this reason it is important to communicate in short sentences using plain language.

Other problems that can arise in interpreted interviews relate to attitudes between the three parties. The interpreter, who should have a completely impartial role, may over-identify with either the clinician or the client (Baker & Briggs, 1975). Concerns that mental health services' clients have expressed about the use of interpreters include the perceived judgmental attitudes of some interpreters, whether interpreters will keep their personal information confidential, and whether what they have said is being translated accurately (Royal Park Corporation, 1994; Pardy, 1995). If a clinician has concerns about the professional behaviour of the interpreter it is their responsibility to maintain professional standards in the interview. The avenues that are open to the clinician include: discussing the issues with the interpreter following the interview; if necessary, terminating the interview; and/or discussing your concerns with the interpreter service.

Employment of bilingual therapists can be a means of overcoming communication barriers, however, it is also crucial that monolingual mental health professionals see themselves as being an important resource for clients who do not speak English. Their efforts may be even more highly valued than they perceive. Working with interpreters is not simple and training for clinicians is important, as is training for interpreters in the area of mental health.

Box 4.1

Working with an Interpreter[1]

It is generally not appropriate to use the patient's family or friends as interpreters. In cases of emergency, the clinician may find that use of lay interpreters is the only way that communication with the client can occur. If this is necessary, staff should try to gain access to an interpreter as soon as possible to verify that accurate communication occurred. Using non-professionals as interpreters may lead to miscommunication, and in certain circumstances, may place clients at serious personal risk and the service at risk of litigation.

Prepare for the Interpreted Interview

Ensure that an interpreter speaks the appropriate language. Often more than one language may be spoken in a country (e.g., a "Chinese" patient might speak Cantonese, Hakka, Hokkien or Mandarin). In some countries many different dialects of a language may be spoken. It is extremely helpful to inform the interpreting service of the region the patient came from in their country of origin. The gender of the interpreter may be an important issue: a female interpreter may be more acceptable than a male or vice versa. Age difference between interpreters and clients may be another important consideration.

How to Conduct the Interpreted Interview

The interpreted interview consists of three stages:
• Pre-interview briefing
• Interview proper
• Post-interview review

---

1 Adapted from Klimidis, Baycan and Punch (2000)

Pre-interview Briefing

It is important to discuss the interview with the interpreter. If working with that interpreter for the first time, it is helpful to explain the setting in which the interpreter will be working (e.g., home, clinic, hospital) and the roles of the staff involved in the interview, (e.g., clinician, ward staff, case manager). It is useful to explain the purpose of the interview (e.g., intake assessment, clinical treatment plan, family meeting). The interpreter should be given the opportunity to advise on what cultural issues may arise during the interview and the patient's possible attitude to the problem or to this form of interviewing. Treat this information as tentative to avoid developing a possibly inaccurate view about the patient and/or carer.

The Interview Proper

Seating should be arranged in such a way to allow eye contact between all parties (although this should not be imposed). A triangular arrangement is usually best. As the mental health worker you should introduce yourself and explain your position and role in this interaction. Particularly if this is the first contact with this patient, to promote trust, explain that the content of the interview will be kept confidential (within the limitations of the law). Ensure that the patient and/or carer understands that the interpreter will also keep interview information confidential. Explain to the patient that the interpreter's role is to interpret all that is said by both parties, and that it is important for each of the parties to pause frequently to allow for interpreting.

In the Interview

When working with an interpreter the mental health worker retains responsibility for directing the interview. During the interview try to speak clearly and use the simplest form of English. Ask questions in a concise and explicit manner. Use brief sentences containing only one idea. Avoid using colloquial expressions (e.g., "Have you felt blue?") especially in phrasing open-ended questions, such as "Where do we go from here?" Pause after a few sentences to allow for interpreting. Long speeches make impossible demands on the interpreter's memory and can lead to distortion or omission of part of the message. Speak directly to the client. In this way the patients feel they are relating with you, and that you are showing interest and concern regarding them and the problems at hand. While interpreters may be able to provide information regarding the meaning and acceptability of behaviour within a particular cultural context, they cannot answer questions such as "Is he psychotic?". This is a request for a clinical opinion. The mental health worker should make a note of instances where something is not understood possibly because of cultural factors. If there is no opportunity to clarify these with the client during the interview the issues may be discussed with the interpreter in the post-interview review.

The Post-interview Review

The mental health worker may want to know more information about certain aspects of the interview. It is important to discuss the interview content and ask questions about impressions or observations with respect to cultural issues. At this time interview process should also be discussed. Were there any communication difficulties during the interview? Were there times when the mental health worker felt a lack of confidence in the communication or confusion related to the interpretation during the interview? Were there important observations made by the interpreter about the mental health worker's communication style, or choice of terms. The post-interview review may also provide an opportunity to debrief the interpreter if distressing issues were discussed in the interview. ■

Translating Psychological Tests and Measures
Cultural Relevance

Many of the issues raised in the previous chapter in relation to clinical assessment also apply to psychological assessment instruments and research measures. If an existing measure is to be translated, the translated instrument should measure the same domain as intended by the original instrument. For example, if it was intended to measure short-term memory in English, it should also measure that in translation, not the person's level of education or literacy (Westemeyer & Janca, 1997). If an instrument is translated directly, it may fail to measure what it was intended to measure, as illustrated by the following case of a crosscultural intelligence assessment:

> A psychologist was asked to assess the intelligence of Melles, a young Muslim man from the Horn of Africa. He came here as a refugee, after having spent his school-age years in a refugee camp where he received little education. He spoke English at a low level of proficiency. The psychologist decided to administer the intelligence test with the aid of an interpreter.

What difficulties might there be, both for the client and the psychologist, in this assessment? If the psychologist uses, for example, the Wechsler Adult Intelligence Scale (WAIS) they are implicitly assuming that intelligence, as measured in Western cultures, is universal. Many questions in the WAIS are, however, heavily reliant on Australian schooling and local cultural knowledge. Some examples from the Information sub-scale illustrate this point.[2] In some African cultures, time may be measured more loosely (e.g., according to the position of the sun, phases of the moon and the seasons)

---

2 Items from the WAIS are not described in specific detail to observe requirements that psychological test items should not be made public.

than in time-driven Western industrial societies (Westermeyer, Janca & Sartorius, 1993). Consequently a question testing knowledge of time reliant on clocks and calendars will be less relevant and, therefore, more difficult for an African client than for an Australian client. Questions regarding local folk heroes, sporting heroes and Australian and British political figures are all reliant on an Australian education and a lifetime contact with local current affairs. These questions too would be more difficult for Melles than for the Australian age group from which the IQ norms were developed. On the other hand, questions relating to Africa and the Muslim religion may be less difficult for Melles than for an Australian client, but Melles probably would not be able to demonstrate this knowledge as he would have failed too many early items to reach these later more "difficult" questions.

The Vocabulary sub-scale also requires education and life experience in the English language. As English is not Melles's first or preferred language, and as he has only limited literacy in his own language, the scale could be more difficult for him than intended. Proverbs, which are included in the Comprehension sub-scale, generally have no meaning in another culture and are often reflective of culture-specific values as, for example, the proverb "a stitch in time saves nine". Questions designed to assess the individual's understanding of the role of various laws or cultural practices in the regulation of Australian society may be incomprehensible to Melles because such laws or practices may contradict Melles's cultural values or even may not have existed in his culture. For example, questions relating to speeding, traffic lights and traffic regulation may be irrelevant to people from cultures where there are few or no cars and no traffic lights (Flaherty et al., 1988).

The WAIS Arithmetic sub-test is dependent on classroom-based learning that is detached from the context in which these skills might be practised in daily life. A psychologist of our acquaintance reported that a Greek woman whom he assessed was unable to complete any of the items in the Arithmetic sub-test. This performance, in the context of the overall WAIS profile, caused him concern that she might be suffering from a neuropsychological disorder. Some time later he came across this woman serving in a greengrocer shop, weighing fruit and vegetables, calculating the cost, and giving correct change. Clearly the WAIS gave a misleading measure of her abilities that she had learnt "on the job" and applied successfully within the context of her routine daily activities. The clinical setting in which psychology tests and other research scales are often administered, and the use of paper and pencil measures may also intimidate people such as Melles and the Greek woman, who may be unaccustomed to such settings and methods (Flaherty et al., 1988).

Test Bias as a Result of Translation

The use of an interpreter by Melles's psychologist will not overcome the lack of crosscultural relevance of some WAIS items. It is not the role of the interpreter to try and infer the nature of the concept that the item was designed to measure and then to convey that in Melles's language. That is the task of bilingual mental health professionals. Even if the content of an item is relevant in another culture, translation can introduce subtle changes in connotation so that a different cognitive domain is being measured than intended (Bontempo, 1993). Translation issues have already been discussed to demonstrate the complexities of assessing depression across cultures. Issues in the translation of cognitive tests such as the WAIS are exemplified by the Similarities sub-scale. This scale asks respondents to describe how two things are like each other. Translated into Greek, this question becomes, "How are these two things physically like each other?" Yet the purpose of the test is to elicit the person's ability to conceptualise abstract properties. To translate items accurately it may be difficult not to provide clues to the answers.

While differences in cultural relevance may change the difficulty level of an item, difficulty may also be changed by translation. For example, the numbers 1–9 are monosyllabic in Vietnamese and Chinese, but in Spanish six of these digits have two syllables. As a result, a digit-span test in a memory scale is more difficult in Spanish than in Vietnamese and Chinese. Bagulho and Chiu (1997) point out that responses to a translated Mini-Mental State Examination can provide a distorted picture of neuropsychological functioning of an individual. For example, items that the examiner choses for the memory test (e.g., pony, ball) may translate poorly from one language to another, or they may represent objects which are unfamiliar in another culture.

In assessing intelligence and other cognitive and instrumental abilities it is crucial to recognise that different societies stress different cognitive processes and abilities. Western culture emphasises information processing and analytical thinking. Other cultures may value agricultural skills, the remembering of stories, or orientation and survival in a harsh natural environment. The Xhosa people in Southern Africa have many words for grass and for methods of carrying (Gillis, Elk, Ben & Teggin, 1982), while the Inuit have up to 49 words for snow (Fortescue, 1984). These subtle distinctions are outside the repertoire of people from Western cultures and they would most likely fail the ultimate intelligence test — the ability to adapt and survive in those environments. The application of Western tests may be irrelevant in some crosscultural contexts. Inevitably, cognitive tests do test the individual's educational and cultural experience and are therefore culture-bound or culture-specific (Flaherty et al., 1988).

The Effect of Translation on the Psychometric Properties of a Scale

For translated assessment instruments to be useful, the terminology in both languages should be equally likely to evoke the same response if put to people with the same symptom (Westermeyer & Janca, 1997). That is, the measures should be psychometrically equivalent (Westermeyer & Janca, 1997). Translation of an item can, however, change any of three properties of a scale:

Translation can change how difficult a scale is to "pass" or to "fail". This has been illustrated by the changes in difficulty of the Information sub-scale of the WAIS, when applied across cultures. Similarly, a scale item may be more or less likely to be endorsed through small changes in meaning through translation. Bontempo (1993) provides an example of this from a crosscultural research study into individualism–collectivism. Item analysis of responses showed that French subjects were less likely than US subjects to agree with the item: "The most important thing in life is to make myself happy". In French this item was translated so that it acquired a slightly different emphasis: "The thing that is most important in my life is to make myself happy" ("La chose la plus importante dans ma vie est de me rendre heureux"). On the advice of a bilingual consultant the item was rephrased so that it was a milder statement, closer in emphasis to the original English and therefore "easier" to endorse: "In my life, the thing that is most important is to make myself happy" ("Dans ma vie, la chose la plus importante est de me rendre heureux") (Bontempo, 1993, p. 160).

Translation can change the range of abilities between which the scale can discriminate. If the difficulty of a scale is increased, then it may fail to make fine discriminations between levels of ability at the lower end of the scale. Alternatively, translation may make the scale "easier" so that virtually everyone can "pass".

Translation may introduce a response bias due to the phrasing of items or response options. Responses may be biased by a need for social approval, by the desirability of a response in a particular culture and by cultural tendencies to acquiesce (Flaherty et al., 1988).

For a test item that has only two possible responses (e.g., "yes" and "no") translation creates the potential for six errors. That is, the "yes" answer can be influenced by any of the three above factors and so can the "no" answer. If the test item has more than two possible responses, then the potential for error increases threefold with each additional response option. If a number of items on a scale are distorted in this way then the mean scores obtained from a scale cannot validly be compared across cultures. Bontempo (1993) showed how item analysis can identify whether changes in difficulty, discriminative power and susceptibility to response bias have influenced crosscultural responses or whether a measure is crossculturally equivalent.

As already suggested, translated items may measure a different cognitive domain than the original item. Scale items generally are intended to measure some latent performance or ability. For example, Melles may have been given a short-term memory test that was designed not only to measure recall, but also concentration and encoding. In translation, items may be distorted and become a measure only of, for example, concentration. As a result, the translated test may not be conceptually equivalent and will be neither a valid nor an accurate measure of memory.

Because cognitive tests are designed to measure specific constructs, it should be apparent that it would not be appropriate to ask an interpreter to translate the WAIS on the spot for Melles. The more apparent disadvantages of this approach are that the interpreter may translate items literally rather than conveying semantic and conceptual equivalence, may convey the correct response, either intentionally or otherwise, and may give the client feedback about their progress.

Etic and Emic Approaches to Developing Tests

To obtain a crosscultural instrument that is conceptually equivalent in all respects (Flaherty et al., 1988), translation of assessment instruments should be undertaken by a panel of bilingual mental health specialists who are familiar with the test domain and with both cultures in question. The test should be translated into the target language (e.g., Amharic) and then back-translated into English by different translators. The two English versions (the original and the back-translated version) are then compared to identify and adjust changes in meaning. This process may require several iterations to remove English idiosyncrasies (Bontempo, 1993). The risk inherent in this approach is that a competent bilingual professional may overcompensate for a bad translation into, for example, Amharic, and produce a good back-translation into English. This will conceal that the translated version of the measure is unsound. This danger can be overcome to some extent, first by having more than one back-translation performed, and second by conducting a pilot-test with the measure in a small population sample (Bontempo, 1993).

The original (usually English) version of a test will have been validated and norms will have been developed for a particular population. The WAIS has age-specific norms that are relevant to a cross-section of the Australian population, but that population will have included few or no newly-arrived refugees from Africa. If a test is to be translated then it should be validated and norms should be developed for the new target population (Baghulo & Chiu, 1997).

To ensure that a measure is genuinely relevant to a culture it may be more appropriate to develop the measure using an emic approach (see chapter 1). Rather than imposing external concepts and categories contained in a translated etic measure that was developed in another culture (Flaherty et al., 1988), a culturally valid measure of the concept of, for example, intelligence may be developed within the culture of interest. This involves investigating what are considered to be indicators of intelligent behaviour, and different levels of intelligence, through consultation with a range of key indigenous advisors and through observation and participation in that culture. Manifestations of various levels of intelligent behaviour would need to be studied over time, and once a reliable set of items has been selected from a wide range of possible items, then norms would need to be established within the local population (Smith &

Bond, 1993). If the emic measure is intended to measure manifestations of psychopathology, then norms would need to be established with normal populations and cut-off scores would need to be determined through further studies comparing patient and normal populations. Comparisons can be made between the emic and etic measures to determine whether these reveal commonalities — "universal" features of, for example, intelligence or depression (Smith & Bond, 1993).

Kinzie and Manson (1987) took an emic approach to developing the Vietnamese Depression Scale (VDS), a measure of behaviours and mood "compatible with the Western concept of depression" in Vietnamese refugees in the United States (p. 192). Bilingual Vietnamese mental health workers listed Vietnamese words describing depressive feelings and behaviours experienced by Vietnamese patients. These items were discussed with the American authors and items were added and/or eliminated if they were not likely to be understood and to take account of the different experiences of rural and urban Vietnamese. A 3-point (rather than the more common 5-point) Likert response scale was used because the bilingual professionals "believed that Vietnamese individuals are less aware of internal contrast than are white middle-class Americans" (p. 193). The selected items were then translated into English by bilingual Vietnamese students to determine if the intended meaning was conveyed. Pre-testing with Vietnamese adults showed that some items needed clarification. The scale was then validated by showing that it effectively discriminated between Vietnamese patients at a psychiatric service and non-depressed community members. The patients all met DSM-III criteria for depression, while patients diagnosed with an anxiety disorder or schizophrenia did not score high on the VDS (Kinzie & Manson, 1987).

Whether an existing etic measure is translated, or whether a local emic measure is developed, the question that remains is, with what populations should normative studies be done? Italian norms for a memory scale developed in Italy may not be applicable in Australia because many of the first generation of Italians who came to Australia in the 1950s and 1960s generally had only a few years of education. At the same time they may have retained the values and speak a version of Italian no longer current in Italy. For these reasons Baghulo and Chiu (1997) have validated and developed Australian/Italian norms for the Mini-Mental State Examination that had originally been translated into Italian and normed for the Italian population in Italy.

When a mental health professional is administering an instrument (whether emic or etic) in a language that he or she does not speak, careful preparation is required and pre-briefing of the interpreter. The interpreter will have to "read" the questions to the client from the questionnaire rather than translating the psychologist's questions. The psychologist in our case study would need to clarify whether she wants Melles's Amharic responses translated back to her in English, whether she or the interpreter is to record the responses, and in what language, and how she will track which question in the scale is being asked by the interpreter. A "dummy" run is recommended to develop familiarity with this rather complex process.

Communication across the language barrier poses particular challenges in both clinical and psychometric assessment. This chapter has aimed to raise an awareness that English mental health terms do not translate literally into other languages and that translation can change connotations in meaning, with associated risks of miscommunication. Equipped with awareness of these issues, clinicians can work collaboratively with interpreters in clinical interviews to communicate accurately and meaningfully with clients who have low English proficiency. Those clinicians who use psychometric assessment instruments will be aware that informal translation of measures raises the risk of distorted results and will explore locating or developing psychometrically sound translated versions of these measures.

Chapter 5

Explanatory Models
of Illness

Key Points

▶ Explanatory models of illness

▶ Sectors of the health
  care system

▶ Stages of illness definition

The Bewitchment of Samuel

In chapter 1 we described the clinical presentation of Samuel, a young
Nigerian man with brain fag syndrome. A distinctive feature of Samuel's
symptomatology was that he believed that he had been bewitched by an
envious acquaintance. He believed that bewitchment had caused his sensations
of insects crawling in his head and various other somatic and cognitive
symptoms. A Western clinician, unaccustomed to supernatural explanations of
illness, may take Samuel's belief in bewitchment as a clear sign of a persecutory delusion. But for people from Samuel's community, the powers of witchcraft provide an explanatory framework for misfortune and suffering
(Fitzpatrick, 1984; Gil, 1998). If a person believes his problems have been
caused by witchcraft, he is more likely to seek help from someone whom he
believes can lift spells than from a mental health service. If he does reach a
mental health service, he may fail to see the relevance of medication that does
nothing to alleviate the effects of spells. In other words, the individual's beliefs
have influenced his conception of the problem (or illness), the help he will
seek, and what treatment he will judge to be relevant to the problem.

Embedded in a culture's belief system are its views on health and illness. In the
same way that beliefs differ across cultures, so cultures differ in the way that illness
is understood. Crosscultural research has demonstrated that cultures vary widely
in the beliefs they hold about the nature of illness, its cause, its mechanisms, its
severity, its course, appropriate treatment and likely outcome (Kleinman, 1980;
Landrine & Klonoff, 1992; Murdock, Wilson & Frederick, 1980).

The next two chapters aim to demonstrate how cultural beliefs influence
conceptions of illness and help-seeking and how differing beliefs can cause a

mismatch between the client's and the clinician's understanding of the presenting problem. To deal with such discrepancies, this chapter aims to provide a framework that will enable clinicians conducting a crosscultural assessment to obtain an understanding of a client's perception of their problem, even if they are not fully familiar with that culture's beliefs and views of illness. The conceptual elements of this crosscultural framework, which will be illustrated by case examples, include:

* explanatory models of illness and how they may be elicited

* the sectors of the health care system in which explanatory models arise and determine pathways to care

* stages of illness definition, showing how cultures differ in their attention to interpretation and treatment of symptoms.

In chapter 6 the influence of a range of cultural beliefs on conceptions of illness and mental illness are explored within the context of this framework.

To provide an introduction to the framework, let's examine the case of Danny. As part of a training session, a group of Australian mental health professionals were asked to consider the case of Danny.[1] They were then asked to answer questions about what they thought were the nature, the cause, the mechanism, the severity, the course, the appropriate treatment and the likely outcome of his problem.

A case example: Danny

Danny is a 22-year-old man who was admitted by the Crisis Assessment and Treatment Team (CATT) to an inpatient unit after he had been reported missing by his parents and found wandering the streets by the police. The assessment found Danny to be very fearful, saying that he was going to die and that he was hearing the voice of a woman making derogatory remarks, and telling him to kill himself. Danny had dropped out of university 6 months ago, unable to sit for his final year medical exams. Since that time he had isolated himself from his university friends and his only social contact was with his aunt and cousin. The family became concerned when Danny said that he needed to kill himself in order to save the rest of the family. Danny has an uncle who was diagnosed with schizophrenia.

---

1 Case adapted from "Mental Health in a Culturally Diverse Society" by I. H Minas, (1990), In J. Reid & P. Trompf (Eds.), *The Health of Immigrant Australia: A Social Perspective* (pp. 250–287). Sydney: Harcourt Brace Jovanovich. Adapted with permission from the author.

Based on this rather frugal amount of information, the majority of the clinicians gave the following answers:

Q. What is the name of the problem?

A. Paranoid schizophrenia was the most commonly suggested diagnosis. Drug-induced psychosis was another possible diagnosis.

Q. What does the problem do to the person? How does it work? What is the pathological mechanism? What caused the problem?

A. Schizophrenia disrupts cognitive, emotional and social functioning. The most likely causes were hypothesised to be hereditary factors (as suggested by the presence of an uncle with schizophrenia); neurochemical imbalances in the brain; stresses associated with loss of vocation; and vulnerability to schizophrenia (associated with his age and sex), the onset of which was triggered by stress. Other causes suggested included witchcraft and the effects of the "evil eye".

Q. Why did it start when it did?

A. Schizophrenia is likely to start in the late teens or early 20s, especially in males. It may be triggered by stresses, such as job loss or educational failure.

Q. How severe is the disorder and how do you know?

A. It is a severe disorder that seriously disrupts social functioning and self-care and is associated with a higher than normal risk of suicide and aggression. Research literature on schizophrenia and the clinicians' clinical experience with clients diagnosed with schizophrenia led them to conclude it was a serious disorder. The problem is not likely to be a brief reactive psychosis because of the lengthy prodromal period, and negative symptoms.

Q. How long will it last?

A. Because of the long prodrome there is a high risk of a chronic life-time disorder, with deterioration of functioning. However, he may have a single episode of psychosis and recover completely.

Q. What treatment is needed? What needs to be done?

A. Initially, observation on the ward is needed to determine whether the disorder is drug-induced. If not, neuroleptic medication should be prescribed and, once stabilised, he should be discharged to the care of a case manager.

Q. What outcome do you expect from the treatment?

A. If the disorder is chronic paranoid schizophrenia, Danny's positive symptoms will be controlled and, with the support of the case manager, he will be able to resume a level of independent social functioning, but not at the pre-illness level. He is at high risk of suicide. If it is not a chronic disorder, he may recover completely, or at a level somewhat below his previous level of functioning.

Eliciting the Biomedical Explanatory Model

The above questions are the key questions suggested by Kleinman to elicit a client's explanatory model of their illness (see Box 5.1, Eliciting Explanatory Models from a Client) (Kleinman, 1980; Kleinman, Eisenberg & Good, 1978). In this instance, the questions have elicited the explanatory models of mental health clinicians, and the answers reveal elements of the over-arching belief system in which the explanatory model is embedded — that of the Western biomedical system. This is the tradition in which the mental health clinicians have been trained. The DSM-IV, which has its foundations in Western biomedical science (as discussed in chapter 1), had strongly influenced the thinking of many of the mental health clinicians in this training exercise. One or two of the clinicians discarded positivist empirical scientific assumptions and suggested supernatural causes such as witchcraft and the "evil eye" to explain Danny's problems. We will return to supernatural explanations later and the reason why some clinicians used such explanations. But on the whole, to explain Danny's problem, the clinicians relied on the scientific research literature they had read, and clinical experience. Because that is the nature of the data that is considered legitimate by the empirical scientific framework (or belief system) of psychiatry (Landrine & Klonoff, 1992).

Popular Explanations of Mental Illness

Generally speaking, the biomedical explanatory model of mental illness is not likely to differ greatly from the popular understanding of mental illness held by lay people of Western background. A lay explanation of mental illness may be less logical and consistent than the professional medical model, but the popular model is nevertheless likely to be strongly influenced by the medical model through contact with the medical profession (Fitzpatrick, 1984; Kirmayer, Young & Robbins, 1994). This more or less shared understanding between the Western client and clinician forms a backdrop that is more likely to facilitate than hinder clinical engagement and treatment efficacy.

People from non-Western cultures, however, are likely to subscribe to quite different illness models arising from different belief systems. When differing explanatory models meet, it is likely, given the status and power of the mental health professional relative to that of the client, that the professional's explanatory model will prevail if the client's explanatory model is not elicited and acknowledged. Failure to do this can have potentially serious consequences, as will be explained after explanatory models have been defined.

Explanatory Models Defined

It is probably already apparent to some extent what is meant when we refer to an explanatory model, but let's be explicit, because explanatory models are sometimes assumed to represent only *causal* explanations. Kleinman (1980) states that explanatory models are a set of ideas about an episode of sickness that are held by patients and by practitioners involved in their treatment. These notions about sickness attempt to provide answers to questions about:

- the cause of the illness
- the time and mode of onset of symptoms
- the nature of the pathology
- the severity and course of the sickness
- appropriate treatment (Kleinman, 1980, p. 105).

Each of these "notions" can be thought of as components of an explanatory model, in which causal explanation is only one component.

All cultures have explanatory models of illness because illness is universally viewed as a disruption of life that requires explanation (White, 1982). But these explanations are culturally shaped and, therefore, show crosscultural variation (Kirmayer et al., 1994; Kleinman, 1980). Lay explanatory models not only "disclose the significance of a given health problem for patient and family", but also they guide choices among available treatments (Kleinman, 1980, p. 106).

Although explanatory models differ across cultures, what they have in common is the creation of meaning; they represent an attempt to make sense of the sickness. By making sense of the illness, the patient and family gain a sense of having some control over the illness, for example, by identifying possible causal agents. If the cause can be established, this in turn often contains implicit ideas about appropriate treatment and healers (Kirmayer et al., 1994; Kleinman, 1980).

As already indicated, explanatory models of illness attempt to answer questions about cause, why it started when it did, pathological mechanisms, severity, course, treatment and outcome. Not all popular explanatory models answer all these questions. Anthropological studies have found that many explanatory models focus on the cause and consequence of illness, with relatively little focus on physical pathological mechanisms (White, 1982). Whatever the extent of the explanatory model, the explanatory model proffered by a client may provide a vital gateway to an understanding of the client's underlying belief system. By asking Kleinman's (1980) questions for eliciting or formulating an explanatory model, and by further exploring the responses, the client's underlying belief system may become apparent. The questions are grouped together in Box 5.1 and phrased as they might be to elicit a client's explanatory model of illness, their expectations of treatment and the meaning of the illness in the client's psychosocial and cultural context.

Alternative Terms for "Explanatory Model"

Other terminology sometimes used in the literature for the concept of explanatory model includes "illness model" (Turk, Rudy & Salovey, 1986), "illness representation" (Leventhal, Meyer & Nerenz, 1980) or "illness schema" (Angel

---

Box 5.1

Eliciting Explanatory Models from a Client

Questions to elicit explanatory models

1. What do you call your problem?
2. What do you think has caused your problem?
3. Why do you think it started when it did?
4. What do you think your sickness does to you? How does it work?
5. How severe is your sickness? Will it have a short or long course?
6. What kind of treatment do you think you should receive?
7. What are the most important results you hope to receive from this treatment?
8. What are the chief problems your sickness has caused for you?
9. What do you fear most about your sickness? (Kleinman et al., 1978; Kleinman, 1980). ∎

& Thoits, 1987). For consistency we will primarily use the term "explanatory model" because of its transparency of meaning and because it is a term that is becoming common in the literature. It also conveys that it involves a cognitive representation or cognitive model of all aspects of the illness experience. The term "illness schema" comes into play during the process of illness definition and will be discussed further when we look at the stages of illness definition.

Disease and Illness

You may have noticed that Kleinman (1980) calls explanatory models explanatory models of illness, not explanatory models of disease. The distinction between the ideas of illness and disease is quite central to an understanding of differences in people's response to sickness across cultures (Kleinman, 1980).

Disease refers to the actual physical pathology and physical malfunctioning in biological and/or psychological processes (Kleinman, 1980; Pilowsky, 1997). The central aim of the biomedical approach is to identify and treat disease (Kleinman, 1980). But the patient presents with more than a disease; they present to a practitioner with an illness experience, which provides a context of meaning to the disease (Kleinman, 1980). "No matter what the nature of the disease and its causes, the disease involves a psychological, social and cultural reaction, the illness" (Kleinman, 1980, p. 78). Illness problems are those difficulties in living that result from the sickness (Kleinman, Eisenberg & Good, 1978). At a personal level, the experience of illness for the individual involves how they perceive and attend to their symptoms, their emotional reactions and cognitive constructions, as well as how they label and evaluate the disease (Angel & Thoits, 1987; Kleinman, 1980; Pilowsky, 1997).

Beyond the intrapersonal experience, illness is also constructed by the way the individual's family, society and culture responds to the disease. This includes the responses of the health care system (Kleinman, 1980). These multiple responses to disease provide it with a meaningful form and explanation, as well as a means (or perception) of control (Kleinman, 1980). Each of these reactions to disease is influenced by culture, which is why "illness is always a cultural construction" (Kleinman, 1980, p. 78). "Illness behaviour is a normative experience: we learn 'approved' ways of being ill" (Kleinman et al., 1978, p. 252). In this context culture may be conceptualised as a means by which disease states are translated into illness. The discussion of neurasthenia in chapter 3 illustrated how culture may influence manifestations or idioms of distress.

The biomedical approach has been criticised for overlooking the patient's illness experience and focusing exclusively on the presumed underlying disease (Kleinman, 1980). How the patient describes their subjective disease experience is of interest to clinicians primarily for the purpose of formulating a diagnosis. In physical medicine the disease can be separated from the illness experience, facilitating control and treatment (Obeyesekere, 1985). Psychiatric diagnosis is based on the medical model of illness, which tends to assume that overt signs and symptoms are directly connected with underlying causes of disorder, which in the case of mental disorders are likely to be located primarily in the brain (White, 1982). But in mental illness there is only a presumed connection between a disease and the subjective experience of the illness (Angel & Thoits, 1987). The "actual physical pathology" of the mental disease usually cannot be verified because its nature is unknown (Kleinman, 1996); "The conception of the disease (i.e., illness) is the disease" (Obeyesekere, 1995, p. 136). A psychiatric diagnosis is an "interpretation of an interpretation", not a direct observation (Kleinman, 1996, p. 19). What the patient reports is an interpretation of the their illness experience, based on their own cultural categories. The mental health clinician makes an interpretation of that interpretation, using cultural categories (Kleinman, 1996), particularly those of the DSM-IV and ICD-10. "Diagnosis is a 'pattern recognition' exercise involving comparison of symptoms with classical patterns" (Pilowsky, 1997, p. 21) that were developed within a Western positivist scientific framework (Kleinman, 1996).

Danny's Illness Experience

Danny, who was introduced earlier in this chapter, was diagnosed as having the disease of schizophrenia. His and his family's illness experience include his increasing social isolation, his personal experience of his "bizarre" symptoms, his understanding of and feelings about these symptoms, the family and relatives' fear, distress and puzzlement at his behaviour, his friends' attitudes towards him, and his discontinuation of studies. The social features, which comprise part of the illness experience, *are* important criteria in making the diagnosis of a disease; they are the parts which contribute to the "pattern recognition exercise" (Pilowksy, 1997, p. 21), but they are often viewed only as information relevant (or irrelevant) to the "predetermined set of criteria" that make up a diagnosis (Cheung, 1995, p. 164). But the course of mental illness is "inseparable from ongoing social events and coping resources" (Kleinman, 1996, p. 19). From the patient's point of view, if only the disease is dealt with by the practitioner, but not the illness experience, then the clinical encounter is likely to be seen as less than successful (Fitzpatrick, 1984).

This description of the diagnostic process may seem an unfair characterisation of clinical practice in Australia. The biopsychosocial model that guides treatment in mental health services does attempt to address the illness experience of the individual (and, ideally, their family) through the multidisciplinary case management system (Health and Community Services, 1994). Optimally, it does this by addressing the individual's needs in the areas of living skills, accommodation, activities, employment and carer support (Health and Community Services, 1995). But these are interventions that follow after a diagnosis is made.

Let's return to Danny and his family to see what their explanatory model might be:

> Danny was born in Australia to Lebanese parents, and is the middle child in a family of five children. Danny had been a successful student at university, sociable and popular. The family reported that things had started to go wrong several months ago. He was spending less time at university and was dating a woman of whom his parents disapproved, as she was of a different cultural and religious background. This had created some conflict at home and Danny had been spending a lot of time with his aunt, Sara, who had a son close to Danny's age. Sara and her son were friends with Danny's girlfriend. Danny's aunt was divorced and non-traditional and due to value conflicts had become estranged from Danny's parents. Danny's parents disapproved of him spending time with his aunt's family, saying that they were a bad influence, and they believed that this aunt was responsible for Danny's deterioration. There had been a lot of family conflict leading up to the admission.

What do you think might be Danny's and his family's explanatory models? And why do you think it matters? Having been provided with this additional information, the group of clinicians who discussed Danny's case earlier pointed to the cultural dynamics in the development of the illness. They suggested that Danny had broken cultural mores by associating with a divorced woman and by disobeying his parents (in a high power distance culture). Both Danny and his family may have seen his problem as retribution for these transgressions, so that none of them saw it as a mental illness. This would explain their delay in seeking help from a mental health service. A small number of the clinicians suggested that Danny's family might believe that Sara has used magic on Danny, that she was a witch, or that she had cast the "evil eye" on him. If the people in Danny's life think that supernatural powers are involved, then how credible are they likely to find conventional psychiatric treatment? Medication may be seen as irrelevant or as potentially harmful and may be rejected. This is why it is important to obtain as full an understanding of the client's explanatory model as possible.

What are the consequences of ignoring a client's illness experience? When the patient, or the family, come from a different culture to that of the clinician the cultural categories used by each to describe and explain the presenting illness may be unfamiliar and incongruent for both, and open to misinterpretation on both sides. The purpose of the explanatory model questions is to elicit the patient's illness experience, thereby minimising the likelihood of misunderstandings. We will return to Danny's case in the next chapter where we will reveal the explanatory model of illness and the associated beliefs held by Danny and his family.

Why Explanatory Models Matter in Mental Health Practice

Explanatory models come into play at a number of stages along the pathway to and within the mental health system. Explanatory models may play a role in delayed presentation to mental health services by ethnic communities; they may lead to misdiagnosis when the client does reach a mental health service; and they may result in inappropriate treatment, and possibly, failure by the client to cooperate with treatment. An understanding of the client's and of the clinician's explanatory model is important in the process of clinical engagement.

Help-seeking

The beliefs and related explanatory models that clients hold about the nature of their problem may be one of a number of factors contributing to the low rates at which ethnic communities use mental health services (Klimidis et al., 1999; McDonald & Steel, 1997; Minas, Lambert, Kostov & Boranga, 1996; Stolk, 1996). Many studies have shown that beliefs about the nature and cause of a particular illness will determine when and what kind of help people seek (Akighir, 1982; Angel & Thoits, 1987; Farmer & Falkowski, 1985; Good & Good, 1982; Sue & Sue, 1987; Weiss, 1992; Young, 1976). If a person does not conceptualise his experience as mental illness there will be a delay in seeking help from mental health services or such help may not be sought at all, unless a crisis occurs (Sue & Sue, 1987). Anecdotally, Australian mental health clinicians report that it is not uncommon for clients from ethnic communities to present to mental health services late in the course of their disorder, and therefore at an acute stage.

Misdiagnosis

If people from ethnic communities delay seeking help until a disorder has reached a severe stage, this might explain findings that non-English-speaking

(NESB) clients, compared to English-speaking (ESB) clients, are more likely to be diagnosed with a psychosis and admitted involuntarily (Klimidis et al., 1999; Stolk, 1996). However, these data also lend themselves to an alternative interpretation. One possibility is that, due to diagnostic error, NESB clients are being over-diagnosed with psychosis when they do present to a mental health service (which does not rule out that NESB clients may present late in the course of their disorder). A clinician's explanatory model is important at this point because it determines what information is taken into account in making judgements about normality and pathology and the nature of that pathology. If a client from a culture different from that of the clinician holds beliefs that are unfamiliar to the clinician there is a risk that these beliefs will be misdiagnosed as evidence of psychosis (Eisenbruch, 1990; Kirmayer et al., 1994; Kleinman, 1980; Lefley, Sandoval & Charles, 1998; Sang, 1996). Misdiagnosis may take several forms. As just indicated:

Culturally appropriate beliefs and behaviours may be misdiagnosed as psychopathology. In a number of cultures it is normative for a person to hear the voice of a loved person who has recently died. A Western clinician unfamiliar with such culturally consistent manifestations is likely to diagnose a client's report of such voices as auditory hallucinations symptomatic of a psychosis (Westermeyer, 1987).

Psychopathology may be misdiagnosed as culturally based beliefs or behaviours. An elderly Indo-Chinese man presented to a mental health service wearing, what appeared to the clinician, to be a Buddhist monk's clothing. He was carrying religious literature and responded to questions in a very philosophical way. He was assessed as having some depressive symptoms but no serious psychopathology. His family subsequently reported that they were concerned at what they perceived to be his bizarre dress and idiosyncratic religious notions. On further evaluation the old man was found to view himself as a reincarnation of Buddha, sent to save the world (Westermeyer, 1987).

The nature of the psychopathology may be misdiagnosed. For example, an affective disorder may be mistaken for a psychosis because the clinician is not familiar with the manifestations of affective disorders in non-Western cultures (Jones & Gray, 1986).

The severity of a disorder may be misjudged. This is best explained by the case example of a South American woman who was admitted to a psychiatric inpatient unit with an acute episode of paranoid schizophrenia. After 10 days her auditory hallucinations and persecutory delusions remitted and her social functioning and personal self-care improved. However, she was not allowed to be discharged because she maintained that she wanted to arrange for a chicken to be sacrificed to repel the curse that had triggered her illness episode. This was viewed by inpatient staff as part of a delusional belief system. Subsequent cultural consultation revealed that this was an accepted folk practice for treating the sorcery that may cause mental illness. While this patient was correctly diagnosed as suffering from a psychosis, misinterpretation of her cultural beliefs resulted in her being detained involuntarily for longer than was necessary.

Research in England and the United States has shown that there are risks of misdiagnosis across cultures because Western clinicians are unfamiliar with the differences in manifestations of mental illness in other cultures (Good, 1993; Littlewood & Lipsedge, 1989). Australian evidence suggesting that there is a potential for misdiagnosis comes from surveys we have recently conducted of the crosscultural training needs of mental health staff in Melbourne. These surveys found that up to two-thirds of 180 staff surveyed rated their knowledge and skills in all aspects of a mental state examination as poorer or much poorer with a NESB client than with an ESB client. Three-quarters of surveyed clinicians also expressed a need for more training in cross-cultural beliefs and understandings of mental illness (Stolk, 2002).

Intervention and Treatment

An important function of diagnosis is to give direction to treatment and other interventions (Minas, 1991). Having made a diagnosis, the clinician's explanatory model determines action (e.g., hospital admission, discharge), treatment and long-term expectations regarding outcome. If misdiagnosis occurs because of crosscultural misunderstandings, then there is a real risk that clients may be prescribed inappropriate or even harmful treatment (Good, 1996b; Minas, 1991), or may be subjected to unnecessary involuntary admissions. Victorian and New South Wales research has shown that hospital admissions of NESB patients are more likely to be involuntary than are the admissions of ESB patients (Klimidis et al., 1999, McDonald & Steel, 1997; Stolk, 1996). Anecdotally, clinicians have reported that a NESB patient may be admitted involuntarily to give the clinicians time "to work out what's going on" with that patient when they do not understand the crosscultural clinical presentation. This is consistent with our training needs surveys, described above, which found a lower level of perceived competence in crosscultural assessments for mental health clinicians.

Clinical Engagement

Risks of misdiagnosis and inappropriate treatment are likely to be minimised if discrepancies between the client's and clinician's explanatory models are elicited and acknowledged. If the client realises that the clinician holds an explanatory model that is different from their own, the clinician may be seen as lacking in credibility and therefore perceived as not trustworthy or helpful. The treatment provided may be seen as irrelevant to the nature of the problem as the client sees it. It would not be surprising then if the client failed to cooperate with treatment or dropped out from treatment. From the clinician's point of view, when a client refuses to cooperate with treatment they are described as "non-compliant", but from the client's perspective, medication may be rejected because it does not address the problem as they conceptualise it. As shown in Samuel's case, resolution of his problem (brain fag) required someone whom he believed possessed appropriate "powers" to lift the spell he was under, not the prescription of psychotropic medications. An ability to elicit a client's illness model and underlying belief system is therefore critical to accurate diagnosis and treatment, which is a basic requirement of ethical practice (Minas, 1998). In explaining their explanatory model, clients may also disclose whether they are receiving alternative traditional treatments. Samuel dropped out of treatment and the clinician did not discover that he was seeking treatment from a traditional healer. However, if she had discovered this, treatment might have been more effective if she had been able to discuss treatment with the healer to negotiate a collaborative approach (Angel & Thoits, 1987). This would enable appropriate Western medical treatment to be provided if indeed he was suffering from a psychosis, as well as showing respect for the treatment that was required by Samuel's explanatory model. In chapter 7, we will demonstrate how to negotiate a shared understanding of the client's problem. This enables the clinician to achieve credibility through their skills of understanding and negotiation, thereby improving the effectiveness of treatment.

Where Do Explanatory Models Come From?

We have described how explanatory models influence pathways to care and treatment effectiveness, but where and how do explanatory models of illness arise? Before people invoke explanatory models of illness, they must first identify and label some changes in themselves as illness (Angel & Thoits, 1987). Kleinman (1980) sets this process of illness definition, and the development and evolution of lay explanatory models, in the context of the health care system. We will first describe this contextual framework of the health care system and then return to place the stages of illness definition in this context. Within the health care system Kleinman (1980) distinguishes the *popular sector* and the *expert sector*, within which are distinguished the *traditional or folk sector* and the *professional treatment sectors* (see Figure 5.1).

The Popular Sector

The popular sector consists of the individual, their family and social networks. "It is the lay, non-professional, non-specialist, popular culture arena in which illness is first defined" (Kleinman, 1980, p. 50). The popular sector is the largest part of the health care system and it is where the major part of illness is treated (Kleinman, 1980; Angel & Thoits, 1987). For example, a cold might be treated with a popular remedy such as a hot lemon drink and honey, with

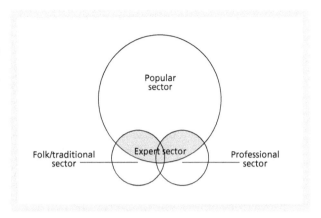

FIGURE 5.1

Three sectors of the health care system (based on Kleinman, 1980, p. 50).

Popular sector

Folk/traditional sector

Expert sector

Professional sector

perhaps some whisky thrown in for good measure. Or an infected cut may be subjected to a poultice that an aunt in the family knows to be effective. A Cambodian parent might treat a child's "wind illness" by "coining", which involves rubbing the skin with a coin. Wind illness or *khyol* is a state of illness in which the body's elements are out of balance (Graham & Chitnarong, 1997). (The need for balance and harmony will be discussed under Asian world-views in chapter 6.)

After home remedies have been found to be unsuccessful, non-Western beliefs about illness causation are likely to lead to treatment being sought from the folk or traditional sector of the health care system, while Western illness causation beliefs are likely to lead the patient to a professional medical practitioner (Kleinman, 1980). However, it is common for treatment to be sought from both sectors, either in sequence, or simultaneously (Angel & Thoits, 1987; Kleinman, 1980; Kirmayer et al., 1994). Treatment received from practitioners also is evaluated in the popular sector (Kleinman, 1980).

Help-seeking

The folk or traditional sector. Folk or traditional medicine consists of the non-professional, non-organised health care sector. It includes a wide range of practices with a blurring between the sacred and the secular (Kleinman, 1980). Shamanism, ritual practices, herbalism, traditional surgical and manipulative treatments, special systems of exercise and exorcism, are just some of the forms of healing (Kleinman, 1980: Sharp, 1994). According to Lefley et al. (1998):

> Traditional healers' skills range from knowledge of appropriate medicinal herbs to modes of negotiation with powerful spirits … [M]ost models of traditional healing, whether for somatic, psychological, social or spiritual ailments, incorporate a supernatural or religious element … [T]reatment typically involves some imbalance in life forces … that can be corrected only

by invoking appropriate counterforces or by ritualistic fulfilment of religious obligations … In treating mental or emotional problems, most traditional healing systems require the intercession of supernatural powers (p. 88).

Kirmayer et al. (1994) argue that folk healers treat the person as an "organic" whole, include the interpersonal and give credence to the importance that violations of values may play in the illness. As discussed previously, value violations were thought to be an issue for Danny as he had disobeyed his family by having a girlfriend of a different religious and cultural background, and by associating with his aunt who was a divorced woman of "bad" reputation.

Traditional healers often do not explicitly elicit symptoms to reach diagnoses or to treat an illness (Good & Good, 1982; Kleinman, 1980). In Iran, astrological information about the patient may be gathered by a prayer writer from family members in the absence of the patient. An illness category may be decided with little information having been obtained about symptoms (Good & Good, 1982). The primary concern of the traditional healer is the treatment of the illness experience (Kleinman et al., 1978). "Healers seek to provide a meaningful explanation for illness and to respond to the personal, family and community issues surrounding illness" (Kleinman et al., 1978, p. 252). While folk practitioners may treat illness effectively, they may not recognise and treat disease (Kleinman et al., 1978). Kleinman (1980) points out that, because anthropological research has focused on sacred healing, relatively little is known about secular forms of healing, and even less is known about the efficacy of either.

The professional sector. The term "professional sector" has generated some controversy as traditional healers also may be considered to be professional practitioners. However, from the perspective of the Western client, the professional sector typically consists of "the organised healing professions", usually modern scientific medicine (Kleinman, 1980, p. 53). In some cultures, however, this may include "professionalised indigenous medical systems" (Kleinman, 1980, p. 54). China has traditional Chinese medicine, India has Ayurvedic medicine and certain Muslim countries have Galenic-Arabic medicine (Kleinman, 1980). In Western countries, scientific medicine has gained professional dominance over all other healing approaches, placing them under medical control and pushing them to marginal quasi-legal status (Kleinman, 1980). Fields of practice affected in this way include chiropractic, homeopathy and naturopathy. Many other health professionals are permitted to practice only as para-professionals under the authority of the medical profession (Kleinman, 1980).

Stages in the Definition of (Mental) Illness and Pathways to Care

As already mentioned, the process of illness definition occurs in the popular sector, and it is during this process that explanatory models are invoked

Kleinman (1980). Angel and Thoits (1987) describe three stages of illness definition, each of which are influenced by culture:

- The pre-symptom stage: when physical or emotional changes are noticed.

- The illness labelling stage: once changes are more persistent and multiply, the individual and/or his or her family may invoke an "illness schema". If the change is evaluated as abnormal then a decision is made whether and where to seek help.

- Choice of course of action stage: a decision is made to seek help from an expert in either (or both) the traditional or professional sectors (Angel & Thoits, 1987).

The processes occurring in each of these stages will be explored in more detail, with a focus on the influences of culture.

Pre-symptom Stage — Attending to Physical, Emotional or Behavioural Change

In the pre-symptom stage, the individual automatically monitors internal sensations in a routine manner, selectively ignoring sensory input that is judged as normal, but paying attention to changes that are not routine (Angel & Thoits 1987). Thus the first step in defining illness involves the individual categorising changes in their physical or mental state as "normal" or "abnormal" (Angel & Thoits 1987). An inference that "something is wrong" is likely to be made when the change in sensations is unpleasant, intense or prolonged (Angel & Thoits, 1987, p. 476). Individuals vary in the extent to which they monitor internal changes. Some ignore them and do nothing while others seek medical attention the moment they become aware of even minor symptoms (Pilowsky, 1997). Excessive attention to bodily sensations that would go unnoticed in most people may be one explanation for psychosomatic presentations (Pilowsky, 1997).

Self-monitoring and evaluation of bodily experiences are significantly influenced by culture and by the individual's "reference groups" (Angel & Thoits 1987). For example, Pilowsky and Spence (1977) investigated reports that Mediterranean patients were more likely to complain of physical symptoms than Anglo-Saxon groups. They found that Greek general practice patients in Australia showed higher levels of hypochondriacal concerns, were more convinced that they had a serious disease, and were less likely to adopt a psychological explanation of their illness than the Anglo-Saxon patients (Pilowsky & Spence, 1977). However, the Greek patients did not show more anger, depression or anxiety about their illness than the Anglo-Saxon patients which "suggests that the alleged 'emotionality' of Mediterranean cultural groups is ... an unreliable guide to the distinctive aspects of their illness behaviour" (Pilowsky & Spence, 1977, p. 450).

Cultural differences in perception, evaluation and response to symptoms may be due to "culturally-specific childrearing practices [that] influence an individual's attention to and interpretation of bodily states" (Angel & Thoits, 1987, p. 476). Gaines (1982) suggests, for example, that suffering is seen as ennobling by people of Mediterranean background; hence they communicate about the ennobled self through a "rhetoric of complaint" (p. 183). This rhetoric would imply a greater attention to bodily changes. But hypochondriacal concerns may also constitute an adaptive response to the stresses of migration and settlement (Pilowsky & Spence, 1977).

There is a risk that cultural differences in attention to somatic changes may lead to stereotyping. An unfortunate effect of such stereotyping is illustrated in the following case:

> A Mediterranean man who was hospitalised in a psychiatric inpatient unit complained constantly of severe headaches. As he frequently tended to complain of various vague physical symptoms, clinical staff dismissed his complaints with the remark that he was Mediterranean. Shortly afterwards he suffered a stroke.

The role of the reference group in defining illness. Whether a physical sensation or mental experience is normal or not is assessed by comparison with the "average health status of one's reference group" (Angel & Thoits, 1987, p. 476). A person's reference group may include the family, work colleagues, friends and/or people in the wider community. The more common an objectively abnormal state is in one's reference group, the less likely it is to be considered significant (Angel & Thoits 1987). For example, certain South American Indians found the absence of a disfiguring skin disease to be so unusual that those in the community who did not have it were considered to be abnormal and had difficulty marrying (Littlewood & Lipsedge, 1989). In many cultures, hearing the voice of a loved person who has died is a normal part of the grieving process (Helman, 1984). As already mentioned in chapter 3, affective states that, in the West would be labelled depressed are considered normal in Buddhist cultures in India (Obeskeyere, 1985). The reference group therefore sets the standard for what are "acceptable" symptoms before a condition is labelled as an illness (Angel & Thoits, 1987). If the disorder is perceived as serious, then help is likely to be sought, unless the disorder is perceived as culturally undesirable, as for example with a psychiatric disorder (Angel & Thoits, 1987).

When the reference group against which an individual is compared is from a different culture, then the potential for misdiagnosis arises. Crosscultural research has found that Eurocentric cultural assumptions contained in many psychiatric and psychological assessment scales reflect the values and norms of the culture in which they were developed (see chapter 4). Consequently, they may distort the mental health status of people from non-Western cultures, so that pathology is either over- or under-rated (Minas, 1996b). African-Americans have obtained higher baseline scores on the Millon Clinical Multiaxial Inventory and on the MMPI, and as a result have seemed more ill than they actually were, according to their own cultural norms (Adebimpe, 1981; Choca, Shanley, Peterson & Van Denburg, 1990). As described in chapter 4, the Self-Reporting Questionnaire distorted the level of depression in an Ethiopian community because the reference group for the SRQ was a middle-class Western population (Kortman, 1987). Research suggests that people from different cultures may differ in the extent to which they are willing to disclose certain symptoms because of perceived stigma or other negative consequences associated with those symptoms (Angel & Thoits, 1987).

Illness Labelling and Evaluation — Invoking Illness Schemata

Once changes in physical or mental state have been compared to the individual's reference group and found wanting, illness labelling and evaluation occurs, still within the popular sector of the health care system. Once abnormal signs start "snowballing", building one upon the other, then the individual or their family are likely to invoke an "illness schema" (Angel & Thoits, 1987, p. 477). The signs will be labelled as a physical, spiritual or mental illness, decisions will be made about its seriousness and home treatment may be instituted. Each of these steps are culturally shaped by values and beliefs (Kirmayer et al., 1994; Kleinman, 1980; Landrine & Klonoff, 1992).

> One of the authors recently recognised how she invoked an illness schema, labelling symptoms and drawing on reference groups. She had a headache that ran in a narrow band from her eye and over the top of her head. The first illness schema she invoked was a sinus infection, which she had had before (self as reference group). When the pain persisted, she thought that the location of the pain resembled that of shingles, a very painful condition that her husband had suffered (family as reference group). A further illness schema invoked was that of a brain tumour! She had read in the newspaper about a mother with a brain tumour who had experienced similar symptoms (community as reference group). Fortunately, the author recovered from her headache the same day.

What is a schema? A schema is a cognitive construct that consists of a remembered organised cluster of knowledge related to a previous experience or object that facilitates (or hinders) information processing (Winfrey & Goldfried, 1986). To illustrate this rather complex definition, consider the illustration on the next page (Figure 5.2); what is it?

The majority of clinicians shown this, admittedly very bad drawing, by one of the authors, guessed it to be a cat, and a few thought it was a dog. No matter. The point is that observers can come up with the interpretation of "cat" because the cognitive schema of "cat" has been triggered by even such minimal information as the sight of a tail, a line drawing, a miaow, or certain letters on a page (D'Andrade, 1990).

FIGURE 5.2

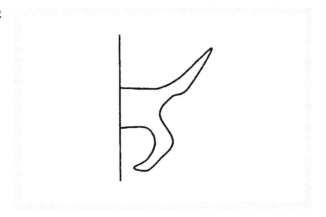

What is this illness schema?

• weight loss

• disturbed sleep

For mental health clinicians, the first likely response is "depression", as the two symptoms are significant criteria for the diagnostic schema of major depressive disorder. We will return to this schema shortly.

A schema is a means of quickly and automatically processing the multitude of information that impinges on the individual (Neisser, 1966; Winfrey & Goldfried, 1986, p. 243). When a person is faced with a new situation or object they are likely to process the information in that situation by matching it to clusters of previously acquired knowledge of similar situations (Juola, 1986; Winfrey & Goldfried, 1986). Such a cluster of knowledge is a schema. Schemata are autonomous and automatic — once set in motion they proceed to their conclusion (Casson, 1983). In this process confirming evidence consistent with the schema will be sought, while evidence not consistent with it is likely to be overlooked or de-emphasised. For example, once an illness schema has been invoked, people will look for additional symptoms that are consistent with that schema, using pre-existing schemata to filter incoming stimuli (Kirmayer et al., 1994; Turk et al., 1986). Thus, a person who attributes her chest pains to a heart attack will start noticing other symptoms consistent with heart problems (Kirmayer et al., 1994). A depressed person may distort and filter information from the environment so that it is congruent with negative self-schemata (Gotlib & McCabe, 1992). A clinician who learns that a new client is suffering from weight loss and sleep disturbance is initially likely to look for further symptoms of the syndrome of depression. While schemata facilitate information processing, enabling the individual to fill in missing data by relying on previous experience, schemata can create risks of misdiagnosis because of their bias towards confirming evidence (Ingram & Kendall, 1986). "Clinicians often observe ... what they expect to observe" (Turk et al., 1986, p. 307).

Many cognitive schemata are socially shared (D'Andrade, 1990). Interpretations made about the world on the basis of shared schemata are experienced as obvious facts of the world. It is implicitly assumed that the information relating to a shared schema does not need to be made explicit, since what is obvious does not need to be stated (D'Andrade, 1990). An example of such a shared but implicit cognitive schema became apparent when one of the authors was feeding coins into her parking meter near work. A visiting Indian Ayurvedic practitioner observed this action with puzzlement and asked what she was doing. She explained that in Australian cities people are expected to pay for using space to park their cars, and that the revenue is used by local government to maintain infrastructure and provide services. He was amazed, as this was not a practice in his city. In Australia when we say, "I'm going to feed my meter", we can assume that our colleagues know all the implicit information about paying for parking space, the risks of being fined, and the purposes of the revenue collected. Our shared cognitive schema obviates the need to make this explicit.

As shown by the earlier example of the sleep and appetite symptoms that elicited the illness schema of depression, diagnostic categories are also a form of shared cognitive schemata. To ensure that a schema does not filter out and distort the full complexity of information available about an individual, it is perhaps even more important to search for evidence that might disconfirm the initial diagnosis as it is to obtain confirming evidence.

Consider this illness schema:

- weight loss
- disturbed sleep
- in a refugee from the Horn of Africa.

The third piece of information immediately increases the range of possible diagnostic schemata such as starvation, posttraumatic stress disorder, a range of physical diseases or, possibly, depression. Obviously, the clinician needs more information to determine which schema fits most accurately.

Choice of Course of Action Stage

Having invoked an illness schema, all of the components of the explanatory model associated with this illness will also be invoked: what the illness is called, the cause, how it works, why it started when it did, how serious it is, how long it will last, what treatment is needed and what the outcome is likely to be. Perceptions of the nature and cause of a problem rely heavily on cultural values (see chapter 2) and belief systems (see chapter 6) and direct help-seeking (Kleinman, 1980; Kirmayer et al., 1994; Landrine & Klonoff, 1992). Folk terms and explanatory models, such as spirit possession or soul loss, "serve to direct attention to specific life events, apportion blame for misfortune and responsibility for illness management, and direct the search for effective help" (Kirmayer, Young & Hayton, 1995, p. 512).

The definition of mental illness may not occur until the individual has passed through several stages of the help-seeking process (White, 1982). If the problem is believed to be due to spirit possession, for example, then a shaman or priest may be consulted. As some cultures do not make an initial distinction between physical illness and mental illness (Landrine & Klonoff, 1992), and because mental health services do not exist in some non-Western cultures (except in the form of asylums), psychological help may not be within the range of treatment options considered. If the person belongs to an ethnic community in Australia and is aware of mental health and psychological services then psychological help may be sought eventually if the symptoms are attributed to personal or psychological problems. But if great stigma is attached to psychological distress, then the problems may be denied, minimised, expressed as somatic symptoms, or contained within the family (Kirmayer et al., 1994; Sang, 1996; Sue & Sue, 1987). It is not uncommon for help for mental illness to be sought from both biomedical and traditional practitioners as each is believed to be able to treat different aspects of the illness (Patel, Musara, Butau, Maramba & Fuyane, 1995).

More will be said about different traditional treatment approaches when we discuss crosscultural belief systems.

Explanatory Models Create Meaning

We have defined explanatory models and explained that lay explanatory models arise in the popular sector of the health system. If we trace explanatory models to their ultimate source, we can also see that explanatory models are embedded in cultural belief systems or world-views, which endeavour to give meaning to life. Elworthy (1989) suggests that in life we are confronted with a whole world of phenomena that baffle human comprehension, and so we search for meaning. As an expression of a belief system, explanatory models of illness may be seen as a means of making sense of the suffering and disruption to life that illness causes (Gil, 1998; White, 1982). When witchcraft or other supernatural forces are invoked to explain misfortune it is as a means of making sense of "things that have no meaning, like incomprehensible ills, adversity, and death, which strike haphazardly and inexplicably return" (Gil, 1998, p. 18). All belief systems, all religions, "provide a vocabulary of suffering", whether this be personal, communal, or even universal (Dein & Lipsedge, 1998, p. 145).

Biomedicine is also embedded in a belief system that endeavours to create meaning. The explanations of Danny's mental illness, which clinicians offered at the start of this chapter, are embedded in a world-view in which there is a prevailing belief in empiricist scientific principles, with an emphasis on logical consistency and replicability (Kirmayer et al., 1994; Kleinman, 1980). This biomedical view has social legitimacy and power. In scientific medicine mental illness is viewed as a discrete intrapersonal disease and the focus is on the biological disease assumed to be underpinning the presenting illness. Medical concepts determine what will be considered relevant data, so that "our methods ... contribute to our results" (Landrine & Klonoff, 1992, p. 273). Working within the biomedical framework of the DSM-IV, for example, the clinician can only ask questions that will verify the model, rather than allowing clients to disclose their conceptual framework. Social and moral problems between individuals, groups and their gods are not incorporated into the model and tend to be discounted or minimised (Kirmayer et al., 1994; Kleinman, 1980). Only natural, observable and verifiable phenomena count as data; ghosts, spirits and imbalances are not considered relevant in interpreting the patient's account of his experience, other than as signs of pathology (Kirmayer et al., 1994; Pilowsky, 1997). It is assumed that "illness can be described and treated without reference to family, community, or the gods" (Landrine & Klonoff, 1992, p. 267).

Limited by the conceptual framework of biomedicine and their professional training, modern health professionals are at risk of regarding "their own notions as rational and to consider those of patients, the lay public, and other professional and folk practitioners as irrational and 'unscientific' " (Kleinman, 1980, p. 57). For this reason, clinicians often find it difficult to deal with a client's cultural values and religious beliefs, interpreting them as primitive, illogical, harmful and in conflict with scientific treatment (Lefley et al., 1998). But the scientific demand for reason and logical consistency is not a demand made by most people (Kirmayer et al., 1994). In lay explanatory models across cultures, logically inconsistent and unrelated views may be held about illness without these inconsistencies being seen as problematic (Fitzpatrick, 1984). "Laymen [and women] are not concerned with their theoretical rigour so much as the treatment options they give rise to" (Kleinman, 1980, p. 93).

An example of how explanatory models can create different meanings from an out-of-the ordinary but observable phenomenon is highlighted in the following extract from the book *The Spirit Catches You and You Fall Down,* by Anne Fadiman (1997).

This account is based on the true story of a Hmong family who took their sick child to be treated in an American hospital and the inevitable clash in values and beliefs that followed:

> Dan (the doctor) had no way of knowing that Foua and Nao Kao had already diagnosed their daughter's problem as the illness where the spirit catches you and you fall down. Foua and Nao Kao had no way of knowing that Dan had diagnosed it as epilepsy ... Each had accurately noted the same symptoms but Dan would have been surprised to hear that they were caused by soul loss, and

> Lia's parents would have been surprised to hear that they were caused by an electrochemical storm inside their daughter's head that had been stirred up by the misfiring of aberrant brain cells (Fadiman, 1997, p. 28).

Both the parents and the doctors want to do what is best for the child, but a clash of cultures occurs as both give a different meaning to the same phenomenon. When a client from another culture reaches a Western mental health clinic, two different explanatory models come together. "One, represented by the mental health practitioner, is derived from a medical reality. The other, represented by the patient, is derived from a cultural and religious reality" (Al Krenawi, 1999, p. 61).

In this chapter we have outlined a framework for understanding conceptions of illness and treatment across cultures. The elements of the framework include the concept of explanatory models of illness, the popular and expert sectors of the health care system, and the cultural influences that bear on stages of illness definition. To illustrate the relationship between explanatory models of illness and beliefs, in the next chapter we will present an overview of a wide range of theories of illness causation across the world. As some cultures do not make the distinction between physical and mental illness, the focus is on beliefs and explanatory models of illness in general, but case studies will be provided that draw clinical implications for mental health practice. This will be followed by a more detailed investigation of two major world-views or belief systems, using the framework developed in this chapter.

Chapter 6

Crosscultural Beliefs about Illness

Key Points

▶ Crosscultural beliefs about illness causation

  ▶ The evil eye

  ▶ Asian world-views and spirit possession

▶ Differentiating mental illness from culturally normative beliefs

The previous chapter examined how different cultures may have quite different explanatory models of illness compared to Western models. These explanatory models can influence when people seek help as well as the sorts of help they seek. Once they do seek help, differing beliefs can cause a mismatch between the client's and the clinician's understanding of the presenting problem. To deal with such discrepancies a framework was proposed in chapter 5 to aid in eliciting and understanding the client's explanatory model of illness. In this chapter the influence of beliefs on conceptions of illness is illustrated by first providing a brief review of a broad range of cultural views on the causes of illness. As previously pointed out, not all cultures distinguish between mental and physical illness; however, case vignettes are used to draw implications for mental health and mental illness. Using the crosscultural framework, two belief systems are examined in some detail, illustrating what implications these beliefs hold for views of health, illness and treatment. We do not endeavour to give a comprehensive exposition of every cultural belief system that clinicians may encounter in their daily contact with clients from other cultures. To attempt this would be to risk oversimplification and the creation of cultural stereotypes.

While it is important for mental health professionals to develop a familiarity with a range of cultural beliefs and views about illness, it is almost inevitable, with the wide diversity of cultures found in Australia, that they will come across people from cultures with which they are not familiar. However, with the tools provided in this and the previous chapter clinicians will be able to elicit a client's and family's beliefs and explanatory models with less risk of stereotyping due to preconceived conceptions of a culture. People vary in the extent to which they subscribe to beliefs commonly associated with a particular culture (Angel & Thoits, 1987), and it is the personal patterning of cultural beliefs that our approach is designed to elicit.

Crosscultural Explanations of Illness Causation

Drawing on anthropological studies of 139 traditional societies across the world Murdock et al. (1978; 1980) developed a classification system of cultural theories of illness causation. Two major categories of illness causation were distinguished: natural causation and supernatural causation. Supernatural causation was further classified into mystical, animistic and magical causation. Further research by Eisenbruch (1990) identified the need for a classification of illness theories prevalent in Asian cultures, which were not included in Murdock et al.'s survey. Drawing on both Murdock et al. (1980) and Eisenbruch's (1990) classification systems, we have distinguished:

- Western theories of natural causation

- non-Western theories of natural causation

- supernatural theories, including mystical, animistic
  and magical causes of illness.

A brief outline will now be provided of the theories falling under these categories.

Western Theories of Natural Causation

These theories include accounts of illness "that would not seem unreasonable to modern medical science" (Murdock et al., 1980, p. 40):

- Infection: invasion of the body by noxious micro-organisms
  (e.g., the germ theory).

- Stress: exposure to physical or psychic strain
  (e.g., overexertion, prolonged hunger, fear, etc.).

- Organic deterioration: physical decline with old age;
  early failure of organs; hereditary defects.

- Accident: unintended physical injury (not supernatural).

- Overt human aggression: wilful infliction of physical injury
  by another person; attempted suicide.

Non-western Theories of Natural Causation

- Imbalance in the qualities of *yin* and *yang* (in Chinese medicine) or *am* and *duong* (in Vietnamese culture).

- Nerve weakness, as in neurasthenia (see chapter 3).

- Loss or blocking of vital energies.

- Loss of vital essences (e.g., *ch'i*), as in semen loss.

- Being "hit" or "caught" by wind; an external wind can enter the body making the person vulnerable to harm by spirits, in turn making them vulnerable to mental illness (Barrett, 1997).

Each of these non-Western theories of causation will be explored further when Asian world-views are discussed.

Supernatural Theories of Causation

Mystical Causation of Illness

An impersonal force automatically causes illness as a consequence of an individual's action or experience, including:

- Fate: illness is due to astrological influences, predestination, bad luck.

- Ominous sensations: particularly powerful dreams, sights, sounds or sensations are experienced and are believed to cause and not just portend illness.

- Contagion: illness is caused by contact with a supposedly polluting object, substance or person (e.g., a menstruating woman; a dead body).

- Mystical retribution: violation of a taboo or moral injunction directly causes illness.

Fate. Anh, a Vietnamese woman, was very preoccupied with her belief that it was her fate to be the wife of a man who had rejected her. To change her fate, Anh returned to Vietnam to visit a Buddhist temple where, she believed, the monk was more powerful than the monk in her temple in Australia. At the temple, the person who wishes to change her fate shakes a stick out of a can containing sticks with numbers on them. The number on the stick directs the person to a wall with numbered holes containing messages about the fate of the person for the coming year. Anh's message predicted a different fate than that she was to marry her former fiancé and her preoccupation with him resolved (T. Dinh, personal communication, December, 2000).

Ominous sensations (1): B.J. Good and M.D. Good (1982) describe a case of fright illness triggered by a powerful dream. A 13-year-old Iranian girl became very ill while she was staying with her grandmother during her parents' absence on holiday. She lost her voice and had severe night fevers. Medical examination revealed nothing wrong and it was suggested her symptoms might be hysterical. The girl attributed her illness to fright she had suffered when she dreamt that her parents had been injured in a car accident and then was nearly struck by a car herself the next day. She believed that this incident confirmed the dream and from that time she had become ill. Following a friend's advice, a brief consultation with a psychiatrist cured her.

Ominous sensations (2). You will also recall the case of Lia, the Hmong girl who was introduced in chapter 5. Western doctors diagnosed her with epilepsy, but her parents thought that she had lost her soul. They thought that this had happened when Lia's sister had slammed the door so loudly that Lia's soul had been frightened out of her body (Fadiman, 1997).

Contagion and mystical retribution. The causes of some illnesses may fit more than one category (Murdock et al., 1980) as shown by the case of an Ethiopian refugee to Israel who was admitted to hospital with a diagnosis of psychosis. She complained of spirit possession and somatic symptoms, including asthma. Her family phoned frequently to enquire about her progress but did not visit her in hospital. For some weeks she was interviewed with the help of an Ethiopian social worker, but it emerged that this worker came from a different part of Ethiopia and understood little of the cultural background of the patient and of the refugee's dialect. When the patient was interviewed in her own dialect it was learnt that she had crushed her baby in a fall during her escape flight. She had carried the baby's dead body for several days, thereby breaking a taboo against touching the bodies of the dead. She was therefore considered impure, both by herself and her family. Staff consulted an anthropologist who advised that contact with a dead body was traditionally considered the most serious form of pollution and required ritual purification in a river in her home country. This was not possible, but an Ethiopian religious leader was consulted, who suggested bathing in the Jordan River for purification. Her symptoms remitted after the ritual (Schreiber, 1995).

Animistic Causation of Illness

Illness is due to the behaviour of a personalised supernatural agent such as a soul, ghost or god.

- Soul loss: Is due to voluntary and prolonged departure of the soul from the body. If death follows from permanent departure of the soul, then less permanent absence logically causes illness. Following the death of a loved one, a person may become so depressed that the soul abandons the body of the grieving person to follow the spirit of the deceased.

- Spirit aggression: Illness is attributed to the direct hostile action of some malevolent or offended ghost, departed ancestor, spirit or god. This is the most common type of supernatural causation because it represents an obvious projection of "overt human aggression" (Murdock et al., 1978, p. 455). Supernatural aggressors include ghosts, departed ancestors, nature spirits, disease demons and deities or gods of varying status.

Soul loss (1). Returning to the case of Lia from *The Spirit Catches You and You Fall Down*, Lia's mother, Foua, explained:

> Your soul is like your shadow. Sometimes it just wanders off like a butterfly and that is when you are sad and that's when you get sick, and if it comes back again, that is when you are happy and you are well again (Fadiman, 1997, p. 100).

For Lia to recover, Foua said that a little Western medicine was needed, because the doctors could fix illnesses involving the body and blood, but they did not understand about the soul; to heal the soul shamanic rituals were also needed. If too much Western medicine was given, that would interfere with the spiritual treatment (Fadiman, 1997).

Soul loss (2). A Hmong woman believed she had lost her soul when she was taken from her flat to hospital by ambulance men. The Hmong community understood her illness in terms of "restless spirits" and that shaman healing was necessary to restore harmony to her spirit. Hospital staff consulted a local shaman who advised that a pig should be killed on the doorstep of her flat so that he could send its soul to bring back the soul of the woman. Permission to kill the pig was refused by government authorities. The woman remained chronically unwell (Zvirblis & Dixon, 1993).

Spirit aggression. In Zimbabwe, an emic study into explanatory models found that mental illness was attributed to a range of supernatural causes, including spirit aggression. The spirit of a person who has been killed by the patient or their ancestors may cause mental illness. Or an ancestral spirit, which has been angered by the disrespectful behaviour of the patient or their descendants, may abandon its protective role and possess the person, causing illness and misfortune. Possessing spirits can only be appeased if adequate compensation is given to the victim or the victim's family (Patel et al., 1995).

Further case examples of spirit aggression will be provided under Asian world-views.

Magical Causation

Illness is due to the covert action of an envious, offended or malicious human being who uses magic to cause injury.

- Sorcery: Is defined as aggressive use of magical techniques by an individual, with or without the aid of a magician or shaman. Sorcery can include verbal spells, prayers, curses, object intrusion, rites, the sending of alien spirits to possess the victim's body and theft of the victim's soul.

- Witchcraft: Involves voluntary or involuntary aggressive action by a human being who is inclined to evil and has special powers. Witches are especially prone to envy and frequently employ the "evil eye" to cause illness. In Zimbabwe, witchcraft is often used because of jealousy at someone's good fortune. The case of Samuel, in chapter 1, is an illustration of this. The evil spirit of a dead person, or birds or animals, may be used to bewitch someone and cause them mental illness, in retaliation for unsettled grievances (Patel et al., 1995).

• The "evil eye": Is a complex and wide-ranging belief system with significant implications for mental health assessment and treatment. The belief system surrounding the evil eye will be presented in the next section.

Western Supernatural Beliefs

Mental health professionals who grew up in a Western culture may prefer to believe that they do not hold any of the supernatural beliefs identified by Murdock et al. (1980) and that they are completely scientific, rational and logical in their thought processes. This view is countered by the Australian mental health professionals who took part in our Crosscultural Assessment Training Program and who conceded with good-humoured embarrassment that they held a range of popular supernatural beliefs:

• No clinicians want a pigeonhole numbered 13 for their mail.

• It is bad luck to walk under a ladder, or if a black cat crosses your path.

• The breaking of a mirror will bring 7 years of bad luck.

• It is not uncommon for people to be reluctant to visit a graveyard at night because they fear encountering ghosts of the dead.

• When passing a cemetery you should hold your breath for fear of breathing in spirits.

• It is common to say "bless you" when someone sneezes; this is to prevent the breathing in of evil spirits, or the sneezing out of the soul.

• The full moon is associated with an increase in psychiatric admissions.

• If someone speaks of having had a run of good luck (e.g., "I haven't had a parking ticket for ages") they should knock on wood to avoid invoking misfortune. This belief is related to the evil eye, as will be explained in the next section.

Crosscultural Beliefs and Their Implications for Illness Perception

In this section a schematic account is provided of two major belief systems or world-views, drawing out their implications for illness and mental illness and treatment. The first belief system is that of the "evil eye", which is a widespread folk belief with an ancient history. The second is not strictly a belief system, but an intertwining of beliefs and philosophies that contribute to Asian world-views, with an emphasis on the belief in spirit possession. The purpose of these accounts is to describe those aspects of a belief system that are relevant to the components of an explanatory model of illness. In addition, attention is drawn to the health care system associated with the beliefs and stages that people go through to reach an illness definition. Bear in mind, however, that not all explanatory models provide answers to all the explanatory model questions; some, for example, focus on the nature, cause and treatment of illness, but may say little about pathological mechanisms (White, 1982).

Alternative belief systems are embedded within a rich and complex historical framework containing diverse views of nature. As already stated, we do not aim to give a complete overview of the belief systems under consideration. It is important for the clinician to realise that the "official doctrine" published in books and other literature undergoes local, family and individual permutations about which only they can tell you. The extent to which an individual or family subscribes to cultural belief systems may also vary with their level of acculturation (Angel & Thoits, 1987). The clinician needs to view each crosscultural assessment as an "individual cultural study". The task in the assessment is to find out the meaning of each aspect of the belief for that person and the person's family.

The Evil Eye

> It is not merely a quaint superstition but a folk belief with serious implications with respect to how individuals perceive the world and their place within it (Harfouche, 1981, pp. 86–87).

Before we explore the evil eye in detail, let's return to Danny and his family, whom we introduced in chapter 5, to discover what they believe to be the cause of his problem, and what treatment is needed.

Danny's parents both believed that his aunt had cast an evil eye on Danny because she was envious of his success in comparison to that of her own son, who was unemployed and a marijuana smoker. Danny's parents were concerned that the treatment being offered in hospital was of no help and, in fact, potentially harmful, so they discouraged him from taking his medication. When they visited him they said prayers over him and gave him a charm in the shape of an eye to wear. Danny's parents wanted him to be discharged immediately so they could take him to Lebanon where they planned to seek the help of a religious healer. They had also made plans for an arranged marriage to take place. Although Danny had been sceptical about traditional treatment before he became unwell, under the influence of his family he cut off contact with his aunt and cousin once he was admitted. He also thought that his sickness was due to an evil eye cast by his aunt. The ward staff believed that Danny's belief in the evil eye was a paranoid delusion and part of his psychosis.

Danny and his family defined his illness (in the popular sector) as being due to the evil eye. They attempted remedies, including prayers and charms, known in the popular sector to be effective against the evil eye. When this was unsuccessful they wished to seek help from the folk sector by visiting a religious healer in their own country. It is not uncommon for folk and religious healers in the country of origin to be seen as having greater powers than healers in Australia. The arranged marriage was a measure to counter the punishment that may have been incurred as a result of the cultural transgression involved in Danny's relationships with his undesirable girlfriend and aunt. The treatment offered by the professional sector (the psychiatric inpatient unit) was not seen as relevant to Danny's spiritual problems and was considered to be incapable of warding off the evil eye. In the discussion of the evil eye that follows, detail is given about the nature of the treatment that would be provided in the folk sector.

The Evil Eye and the Perception of Illness

Modern literature on the evil eye is scarce and in the field of health and mental health it is practically non-existent. We will provide an overview of the evil eye, drawing out its implications for general health and mental health. This account illustrates first how beliefs influence understandings of illness and mental illness, and second, how folk belief systems such as the evil eye are more complex, multidimensional and widespread than those not reared with these beliefs may realise. Forms of belief in the evil eye can be found almost universally. It may be tempting to regard beliefs that are different to one's own as irrational or superstitions, but these superstitions may actually be systems of belief embedded in thousands of years of history and culture. Efforts to treat or correct them may only cause the person who holds these beliefs to conceal them. What science regards as irrational may be an aspect of experience that exists closer to home than may be comfortable. You may recall that, early in this chapter, one or two of the clinicians who attended our training program suggested that Danny's problem was caused by the evil eye. The clinicians who suggested this either grew up in a culture where there was a strong belief in the evil eye, or had encountered clients who held this belief.

This account of the evil eye contains answers to most of the questions that clinicians should ask to elicit an explanatory model. With this account we want to alert clinicians to how extensive a belief system can be.

Evil Eye — Definition and History

To fully appreciate the health and illness implications of the evil eye, it is important to have an understanding of some of its underlying principles and history.

Dundes (1981) provided the following definition of the evil eye:

> The evil eye is a fairly consistent and uniform folk belief complex based on the idea that an individual, male or female, has the power, voluntarily or involuntarily, to cause harm to another individual or his property merely by looking or praising that person or their property. The harm may consist of illness, or even death or destruction (p. 258).

According to Dundes (1981, p. 266) the evil eye belief complex has its origins in "a number of interrelated folk ideas found in Indo-European and Semitic world-views". The first idea is that life depends upon liquid. This is based on the concept of the "water of life" and refers to semen, blood, milk, saliva, bile and other bodily fluids. The underlying principle is that liquid means life while loss of liquid means death. Wet and dry are an oppositional pair as are life and death. The second idea is based on the belief that "there is a finite, limited amount of good health" and wealth in existence and consequently "any gain by one individual can only come at the expense of another". The third is that "life entails an equilibrium model" such that if someone possesses "too little wealth or health" then these individuals constitute a threat to those with "sufficient or abundant wealth and health". Each of these principles have implications for fortune and misfortune and for good and ill-health, as will become apparent as questions for eliciting the explanatory model of the evil eye are answered below.

References to the evil eye can be found in the oldest monuments in the world, particularly in ancient Egypt, providing testament to the historical significance of this belief (Dundes, 1981; Elworthy, 1989). The evil eye is mentioned in the literature of every land since history began to be recorded. Neither science nor religion have been able to shift this fixed belief (Elworthy, 1989). The evil eye is often thought to be unique to Mediterranean cultures, but it is a much more widespread belief that can be found in countries as wide-ranging as India, Iran, Turkey, Greece, Italy, Roumania, Vietnam and the countries of the African continent.

According to Woodburne (1981, p. 56), "The evil eye is very common in India, being recognised even in the sacred books of both Hinduism and Islam. It is a Hindu belief that the eye gives forth the most powerful of all emanations from the body". The possibility of transferring evil from one person to another by sight is commonly held. The victim may not always realise when the evil eye is being cast, "for even a look of admiration may be a cloak for it".

The belief is also held with deep conviction in Iran and has the greatest influence of all of the superstitions. The history of the evil eye is found in ancient Zoroastrian literature and later in the Koran (Donaldson, 1981). In the Koran there is reference to the evil eye in connection with the prophets. It is said that when a woman tried to harm Mohammed with an evil spell, four promises or prayers (*surahs*) were revealed to him so that he might not fear, but rather place his trust in God. These four surahs are considered most efficacious against the evil eye and are written and worn by people who think they have fallen under the spell of evil, or they are read repeatedly until the effects of the eye are removed (Donaldson, 1981).

Another account is given in the Koran of a woman who asked the Prophet Asma if she could use a spell for a family affected by the evil eye. The Prophet replied, yes, for "if there were anything in the world which would overcome

Fate, it would be an evil eye" (Donaldson, 1981, citing the Koran, Reply from the Prophet Asma, p. 67).

Anglo-Celtic cultures have also been influenced by the belief in the evil eye. For example, in England at the time of the Black Death it was believed that even a glance from a sick person's eyes could infect those upon whom the glance fell (Dundes, 1981). Prevalent also in modern English are phrases such as "the eyes are the window to the soul", "the mother's loving gaze" and the "dirty look". These are references in the English language that suggest that the eyes communicate something other than that which can be put into words and imply why the eyes are of such significance across cultures.

The Evil Eye as an Explanatory Model of Illness

In this section, clinical implications of belief in the evil eye are illustrated through answers to explanatory model questions.

What is it called? The evil eye, *jettatura* (in Italian), *mal de ojo* (in Spanish).

How does it work? In many cultures, people know what is meant by the evil eye, but not all agree how its power is exerted. Some say that the power of the look alone is enough, others say that words must accompany the look to make it really dangerous. There are several different accounts of the nature or operation of the evil eye, and three of these will be described: evaporation, fascination, and the ghost theory (Brav, 1981).

According to the theory of *evaporation* a malignant influence from the eyes of an envious or angry person infects the air and can penetrate the body of someone or something else. The eyes are believed to be porous, allowing waste products, which are in the form of a poisonous vapour, to evaporate. The eyes, as the window to the soul, allow for even a glance from an envious person to contaminate the air (Brav, 1981; McCartney, 1981).

The theory of *fascination* is based on mesmerism, hypnotism or bewitchment in which the eyes capture the gaze of another who comes under a spell.

The *ghost theory* is based upon the belief that "numerous evil spirits exist in the eye which, on certain occasions, under provocation, may do harm to others, cause disease and even death" (Brav, 1981, p. 50). The ancient Jews were believers in ghosts and many modern-day Jews still believe in evil spirits that are able to be transmitted by the evil eye. "It is highly probable that the practice among the Jews of covering the eyes of the dead with pieces of porcelain is to guard against the evil spirits hovering in them" (Brav, 1981, p. 50).

What causes it? That the evil eye is common to all societies has been linked to the idea that it is rooted in envy and jealousy, which is a universal factor in human societies (Elworthy, 1989). Envy is not just about malevolence but also about love: a loving gaze has the power to invoke the evil eye. Envy and love are not necessarily opposites; they can coexist. "Love is of the same origin as disease, which through sight strikes passion into the soul" (Elworthy, 1989, p. 33).

Remarks about an individual's wellbeing are tantamount to praise of one's health, and are feared in many parts of the world (McCartney, 1981). Somali mothers cringe when doctors tell them their babies are big and healthy, out of fear that the evil eye will cause something bad to happen to the child (Lewis, 1996). More familiar to some people are references to the danger of good fortune in the English language, such as "touch wood" or reference to someone else's good fortune, for example, "he's riding for a fall". These references are consistent with the principle that there is a finite, limited amount of good health and good fortune in existence.

The danger of *praise* is thought to come from three sources: "(1) the inadvertence or the ignorance of well-meaning people who let slip complimentary remarks; (2) the envy and malevolence of those who have the evil eye; and (3) the jealousy of the gods, who permit no mortal to be supremely beautiful, happy or prosperous without paying" (McCartney, 1981, p. 10). Although the evil eye is generally seen to be involuntary, if a loving gaze can unwittingly cause danger then it follows that the effect would be more severe if the gaze is cast with some malevolent intent.

In different cultures there are varying accounts of how someone might be predisposed to be a bearer of the evil eye. In Roumania, for example, the evil eye is thought to be borne by persons with blue or green eyes; with eyebrows that meet; those who have been weaned twice over; and those born with a caul (the membrane that encloses a foetus and is sometimes found on a baby's head at birth; Brown, 1993; Murgoci, 1981). In Lebanon, the evil eye is often thought to belong to an envious woman who possesses what is called an "empty eye". She is usually not aware of the effect of her eye, or if she is, cannot help it. Such a woman may be a neighbour, friend, relative, a childless stranger or even one with a poor milk supply. Boasting or bragging about a good milk supply by the mother or relatives can invite the evil eye; in-laws or other trouble makers in the family may cause the milk to dry up through their envy or dislike of the lactating mother (Harfouche, 1981).

In India, the bearer of the evil eye is likely to be a person who is suffering from some physical defect and who could therefore cast an evil eye on a person with a healthy body. An evil eye gets its evil character from the person's own potentiality. The eye is that part of the person through which the evil influence is transferred (Woodburne, 1981).

In Iran, the possessor of an evil eye may or may not know he or she has it. It can be related to the sign of the zodiac into which a person is born, or it can be caused by a star that was rising at the time of birth. Numerous stories are told about the effects of the evil eye, about sickness and death befalling those who have come under its influence. In fact, when someone is ill it is common to try and work out whose eye harmed them (Donaldson, 1981).

What does it do to the person? The effect of the evil eye has a negative impact on a person's health and wellbeing, making those who are most beautiful, healthy and prosperous vulnerable to its effects. A typical syndrome includes symptoms such as loss of sleep, headache, constant yawning, digestive problems, fever, depression, general weakness, even death. In Turkey and Lebanon, for example, it has been associated with emotional and mental distress and illness. In India it is also associated with the destruction of animals, gardens, crops and buildings. There are many accounts of its impact on babies and infants as well as lactating mothers. This is particularly prevalent in the Middle East (Harfouche, 1981; Woodburne, 1981; Donaldson, 1981).

Harfouche (1981) provides an account of the consequences of the evil eye on lactating mothers in Lebanon. The effect is sudden and immediate: the milk supply decreases, stops or changes, the breasts may become painful and the mother may get sick and develop a fever or lose weight. The evil eye may also affect the health of the infant. The onset of disease associated with the evil eye is often sudden and dramatic; prior to its effect the infant has no complaints and appears to be in perfect health. Illness can include convulsive seizures, severe spells of crying, refusal to nurse, colour changes, gastrointestinal tract symptoms, and sudden death (Harfouche, 1981).

What kind of treatment is needed? It can be important for clinicians to have an understanding of treatments for the evil eye as some of the practices may be incorrectly interpreted as bizarre behaviour and as evidence of delusional beliefs and psychosis.

Treatment for the evil eye generally aims for both prevention and cure, and the two aims are usually inextricably linked. Treatments frequently combine both witchcraft and religious practices (Harfouche, 1981). The witchcraft component has similar patterns across cultures, whereas the religious devices differ according to an individual's religion (e.g., Islam; Christianity; Hinduism; Judaism). Figure 6.1 schematically sets out the contributions of the different components to treatment and the extent to which they overlap. Each of which will be explained more fully below.

Treatment for the Evil Eye

The religious components of treatment include praying, wearing and displaying religious pictures to ward off the evil eye, sacrifices and the visiting of holy places believed to have healing powers, such as sites of ancient churches, temples, springs, fountains or caves. If praying is done by men of religion, such as *hodjas* in Turkey or priests in Greece, it is believed to be more effective. In Greece a prayer may be read over the sufferer using oils from sacred lamps.

The witchcraft component is based upon two fundamental principles that constitute the roots of magic. First are devices based on the law of similarity, which may be termed "homeopathic, or imitative magic" whereby "like produces like" (Harfouche, 1981, p. 94). Second are devices based on the law of contact, or contagion, which may be termed "contagion magic", each of

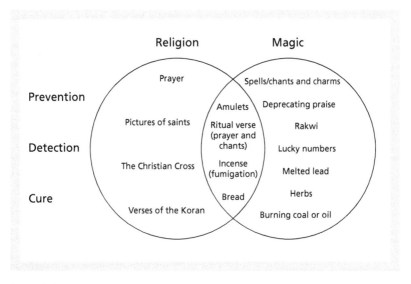

FIGURE 6.1

Overlap between religion and magic in the prevention, detection and cure of the evil eye.

which holds that things that have once been in contact continue to act on each other (Harfouche, 1981, p. 94).

There are rituals for both positive and negative magic. Positive magic says "do this in order that 'so and so' may happen". Charms and amulets are examples of the positive precept in magic. Negative magic prohibits: "do not do this, lest 'so and so' should happen", and taboos are a negative applications of magic (Harfouche, 1981, p. 84).

Verbal invocations. What is said, as for example in verbal invocations, has a fundamental role in treatment. In religion, verbal invocations involve more than just prayer, as many languages and cultures have ritual religious sayings that are evoked by praise. An Irishman would not receive a compliment without responding "Glory be to God", and a rural Englishman without "Lord be with us" (Elworthy, 1989). Implicit in these rejoinders is the belief that acknowledgement of a higher protective power averts the danger of fascination. This, and not gratitude, is likely to be the motive. In Arabic, ordinary conversations are interspersed with *Ma' sha'llah* and *In sha' llah,* meaning "what God wills" and "if God wills". People use these expressions to protect themselves against the evil that "may lurk behind a remark of appreciation or admiration" (Donaldson, 1981, pp. 66–67). If, in conversation, someone says, "So I'll see you next week", an appropriate response would be, "If God wills". If someone enquires after the health of another's children the response will require more than a "Good, thank you", it would require "Good, thank God", at which point the person who asked will respond with "May God bless your children". Another example is, if someone has cooked a good meal it would be appropriate to say, "The food is delicious", followed immediately by, "May God bless your hands".

Magic also makes use of verbal invocations, with spells, incantations and rituals, lucky numbers, provocative verbal formulae, and disparaging or belittling remarks. The custom of using deprecation after praise, as well as concealment of good fortune, is common across many cultures. The parents of an attractive or bright child may refer to the child as ugly or stupid, or give her the name of a domestic animal such as "donkey" in order to keep the child from being harmed. If a precocious child has done intelligent or amusing things, the very superstitious mother will spit upon the child. Spitting is believed to overcome the evil consequences of admiration, for the Prophet spat on Ali when he sent him forth to fight demons (Donaldson, 1981). Another example is of a Macedonian woman who took her new baby to visit relatives. One of the relatives exclaimed, "What a beautiful baby, I hope a chicken shits on her nose." Similarly, in Hebrew, protective measures are contained in ritual phrases (Brav, 1981).

Amulets. Amulets are very commonly used to both prevent and treat the evil eye. Dating back to ancient Egyptian times, amulets are meant to protect the person wearing them from harm. An amulet can be anything worn against the person as a charm with the intention of averting evil, mischief, disease or witchcraft (Elworthy, 1989). They have significance in both religion and witchcraft. Amulets have been and are still part of many other cultures and appear in different forms. One form of modern amulet is the Cross, which has taken on religious significance in Christianity, however, it is also a symbol dating back to ancient Egypt (Elworthy, 1989).

In Lebanon commonly-worn amulets include the blue bead and the horseshoe, which is symbolic of the crescent or the waxing phase of the moon. The moon (and its phases) is important to the Lebanese because it is believed to affect not only agriculture, but also mood, behaviour, sanity and insanity. With the changing cycles of the moon the sane may become jittery and the insane agitated and out of control. The hand of Fatima is another common Lebanese charm, as well as a glass eye, or a piece of wood (Harfouche, 1981).

The Iranians use a number of protective devices, including prayers and amulets, the most common of which are shells, stones, mother-of-pearl and various parts of animals (Donaldson, 1981). In Greece amulets include beads, garlic, eyes and horseshoes. In Turkey and other Islamic cultures, the amulet is a small scroll upon which particular prayers (surahs) from the Koran, as well as ritualistic signs and numerical configurations, are inscribed by the hodja. The scroll is folded into a cloth of various colours or leather, and is worn as a necklace or fastened to the person's clothing with a safety pin under the arms or over the chest. It is believed that the amulet will protect the person against the *jinns* and other spirits that are believed to cause mental illness. Amulets are an expression of a widespread belief in the power of written material, particularly when it is from the Koran.

Other treatments. In addition to amulets there are a number of other commonly used treatments for the evil eye. Fumigation is one of these and involves the burning of incense in sacred places. This is based on the following ideas: that it pleases God and therefore is capable of repelling evil; burning has a purifying effect; the fumes obscure the path of evil and so deter it; evil is incompatible with the pleasant scent of incense (Harfouche, 1981).

Another form of treatment is *rakwi,* which involves reciting an incantation or prayer over a liquid medium in a vessel over the head of an affected infant, which the infant later drinks. The incantation or secret prayer for performing rakwi is known to only a few people in the community, usually women (of the Sunni or Druze religions), who yawn several times whilst reciting the incantation. If the performer sheds tears over the liquid while yawning it is a strong indication that an evil eye has been cast on the infant. Another form of rakwi is *sakbeh,* which consists of melting a piece of lead in a spoon while saying a prayer. Once the lead is melted, it is poured into a small vessel containing water, which is then held over the head of the afflicted infant. Upon the melted lead reaching the cold water it solidifies in the shape of an eye, a face, or some other features of the suspect (Harfouche, 1981). In Greece, oils in water are used in a similar way: if the oil mingles with the water an evil eye is confirmed and nothing more needs to be done (Hardie, 1981).

In Iran the suspect may be detected by recalling the last person with whom the affected person was in contact. Steps can then be taken to detect the guilty person, for example, by holding an egg between two palms and placing pressure upon it as the name of each suspect is spoken. At the name of the guilty person the egg will break (Donaldson, 1981). Suspicion is directed towards those who are considered to have a reason for being jealous, such as the mother of a sick child who has seen someone else's healthy child.

The evil eye healthcare system. The evil eye belief operates within its own traditional or folk health care system, which lies outside the professional medical sector. Western researchers and health practitioners have been concerned about delays before treatment is sought from the modern professional health sector. An example of this is provided by a Lebanese study into child and maternal health, conducted at the American University in Beirut (Harfouche, 1981). Interview and questionnaire data were obtained from 379 expectant mothers of different ethnic and religious groups such as Armenians, Maronites (Christians) and Sunni (Moslems). Many aspects of infant care were considered and the evil eye was included because it was seen to have an undeniable influence in the maternal nursing situation. Demonstrating the mothers' ambivalence towards the evil eye, the study found that 55% of the mothers acknowledged that they believed the evil eye could harm their infant and affect milk supply, but 100% of the babies were found to be wearing amulets or charms, either pinned over the shoulder or hung on a golden chain around the neck or wrist.

The evil eye is seen as a critical factor in maternal care in Lebanon. These mothers saw physicians and other health workers as ignorant of the illnesses caused by the evil eye and useless at counteracting it. In seeking treatment, evil eye repellents are sought before medical advice is sought. Medicines prescribed by physicians are not seen to help, and if the evil is not detected and repelled immediately then it may cause sudden and severe illness, disability or death (Dundes, 1981).

According to Harfouche (1981) the art of healing illnesses caused by the evil eye is a reality in the lives of the Lebanese mothers. "It is an institution with ardent advocates and sponsors who uphold its established concepts and practices" (p. 93). The evil eye operates within its own health care system in which the role and characteristics of each person is defined. These include: the suspect, the patient, the diagnostician and the druggist (Harfouche, 1981).

The *suspect* is the envious person who exerts ill-effects on others by a look or an expression of envy.

> The *patient* is the envied healthy, handsome child. The *diagnostician* is the shrewd and experienced one who inspires confidence and is endowed with special insight. Like the physician, the diagnostician is also a healer or a performer who counteracts or removes the evil effect with drugs once the diagnosis has been made (Harfouche, 1981, p. 93).

"The *druggist* dispenses herbs, incense, lead, charms and special preparations in correct proportions" (Harfouche, 1981, p. 93). Like Western pharmacists, druggists operate shops from which they make a living. There is an informal type of schooling in the practice that is transmitted within a family circle (e.g., sons and daughters learning from their parents).

> Like Western medicine, the art of healing the evil eye has preventative and curative aspects. The devices used in each case depend upon a proper understanding of the cause, effect and mode of transmission by an intelligent specialist with adequate training and perseverance in his art (Harfouche, 1981, p. 93).

The evil eye belief is not one that can be ignored or easily argued away in an attempt at re-education through psychoeducation, using the Western explanatory model. Its power needs to be understood, respected and worked with as part of the therapeutic process in any health or mental health setting. Let's see how this process was undertaken with Danny and his family:

> Danny was reviewed by a new Arabic-speaking psychiatric registrar who was familiar with the evil eye belief complex. She explained the belief complex to the team as well as the importance

of negotiating treatment. The registrar and the ward staff spent some time with Danny and his family discussing their beliefs and explaining the treatment they were offering. Once the family had gained some trust in the treating team they were less suspicious about the medication and agreed to encourage Danny to take it. The family also agreed to postpone their trip to Lebanon until Danny was considered by the doctor to be well enough to travel.

The strategy used by the psychiatric registrar is a good example of the process involved in negotiating explanatory models, a process that will be more fully explained in chapter 7.

Asian World-views
Distinguishing Culturally Sanctioned Beliefs from Psychopathology
The following case illustrates a number of practices and beliefs associated with Asian world-views, which will then be elaborated:

A Case Example of Spirit Possession: Hong

Hong is a married Vietnamese woman in her 20s who has lived in Australia for three years. She completed high school in Vietnam. She is living with her husband and his parents and is expected to help in the family grocer shop. She has an unhappy marriage, is socially isolated, and speaks little English. Hong practises the Buddhist faith. A mental health Crisis Assessment and Treatment Team was called by police after they discovered her late at night on a freeway overpass, holding her 18-month old son, and looking distressed.

Hong told the CAT Team that she was possessed by the spirit of her dead sister who died in a drowning accident at the age of 15. Her sister's spirit was wandering the world restlessly, seeking a place to settle. She thought her son was also possessed, as his skin felt cold, as if he were dead, and his body sometimes grew large and distorted. Sometimes when she was doing the washing the water seemed to turn red, as if it were blood. She acknowledged that she had had thoughts of jumping onto the freeway with her son.

The family reported that Hong sometimes spoke to her sister's spirit and sometimes in the voice of her sister's spirit. They had taken Hong to a woman to be treated for spirit possession some months before. This woman told them to make food offerings to the ghosts. The family was instructed to burn fake money around her and to make her drink liquid containing ashes in it. The family agreed that ancestral ghosts were in the house. Hong herself also made offerings to the ghosts by placing offerings of rice and other food in front of a shrine. When the CAT Team visited the house, they found that almost the whole floor of the front room was covered with these offerings.

The family said Hong often complained of headaches and wanted to leave the house to relieve the headaches. Recently, when her husband tried to stop her leaving the house, she threatened him with a knife.

Hong resisted being admitted to hospital, but when the CATT medical officer asked the sister's spirit permission to treat Hong, the spirit agreed. On admission she was reported to be suffering from persecutory delusions, delusions of control and as having auditory and visual hallucinations. She was treated by an Asian psychiatric consultant who did not prescribe medication, but chose to observe her progress. Hong recovered fully within three days with a discharge diagnosis of brief psychotic disorder.

This case illustrates the complexity of distinguishing beliefs that are culturally accepted from psychopathology. Hong clearly has a number of personal and social problems associated with migration, resettlement and family conflict that may have triggered a brief psychotic disorder. However, spirit possession is culturally sanctioned, as will be discussed shortly, and the family agrees that ghosts are present. On the other hand, symptoms, such as her son's body seeming enlarged and distorted, seem atypical and not consistent with the family's beliefs. Moreover, Hong has demonstrated risk behaviours, including an apparent plan to jump onto a freeway with her child, and threatening behaviour towards her husband with a knife. On balance, it would appear that she may indeed be suffering from a psychotic disorder. The perception that the washing water sometimes turned red suggests that posttraumatic stress disorder should not be ruled out as she may have suffered traumatic experiences during or after the Vietnamese war. However, as she recovered so quickly, brief psychotic disorder appears to be the appropriate diagnosis, and would be consistent with World Health Organization findings that single acute psychotic episodes are more common for people from developing than from developed cultures (Jablensky et al., 1992).

The fact that spirit possession featured as part of Hong's condition serves as a reminder that cultural beliefs may influence the content of psychotic delusions and hallucinations (Westermeyer, 1987). In Western culture, delusions are likely to feature flying saucers, computers or electronic spying and listening devices. The extent to which the beliefs exceed culturally sanctioned boundaries and become abnormal can be ascertained by asking other family members or cultural consultants. Hong's offerings to the spirits, for example, far exceeded normal practices, according to her family.

Although the belief that one is possessed by spirits is normative in many parts of the world, and is not considered a sign of mental illness:

> ... that is not to say that spirit possession is normal, in the sense that most people expect to be possessed during their life. Rather, *it is a culturally specific way of presenting, and explaining, a range of physical and psychological disorders* in certain circumstances ... Possession, then, is an abnormal form of behaviour, but one which is in conformity with cultural values, and the expression

of which is closely controlled by cultural norms. These norms provide guidelines as to who is allowed to be possessed, under what circumstances, and in what way, as well as how this possession is to be signalled to other people (Helman, 1984, p. 217, emphasis added).

Some of the practices described in Hong's case, such as the burning of paper money, will be explained in the account of Asian world-views. One further observation to make on this case, however, is to note the culturally sensitive intervention employed by the medical officer when he asked for permission to speak to the sister's spirit. By acknowledging the reality of the experience of possession for Hong, rather than dismissing this as psychotic behaviour, he was able to initiate the process of negotiating explanatory models and treatment. More will be said about this process of negotiation in the next chapter.

Asian World-views and the Perception of Illness

As already explained, we have not called this section "the Asian belief system" as no one belief system prevails in Asian cultures. Rather, a number of major beliefs and philosophies intertwine in such cultures as those of China, Indo-China and Japan, which contribute to Asian world-views. These world-views "underpin the expression of health and illness" (Kleinman, 1980; Lock, 1982; Luntz, 1998; Phan & Silove, 1997, p. 86). Included in these world-views, with local variations and emphases, are:

- Buddhism
- the Cult of the Ancestors
- the philosophy of Confucius
- the philosophy of Taoism
- Christianity
- supernatural beliefs (Kleinman, 1980; Luntz, 1998; Minas & Evert, n.d.).

Each of these beliefs and philosophies (with the exception of Christianity) will be discussed in turn, drawing out their clinical implications.

The primary source of these religious and philosophical traditions is Hinduism, which can be traced back 3500 years (Scott Littleton, 1996), providing testament to the antiquity of the belief systems under discussion.

Buddhism

Buddhism is the great "daughter religion" of Hinduism, and was first preached in northern India in the late 6th century BC (Scott Littleton, 1996, p. 9). In its process of expansion across Asia in various forms, Buddhism became a transcultural religion, managing to coexist with indigenous beliefs and practices, including the Chinese traditions of Confucianism and Taoism (Scott Littleton, 1996).

Aspects of Buddhist doctrine relevant to illness include the Four Noble Truths, which incorporate the Eightfold Path to the Cessation of Suffering (*Duhka*) (Rotem, 1996). According to Buddhism, the fundamental problem of human existence is the fact of impermanence — no happiness can last forever and there will always be suffering and death. The first goal of Buddhism is acknowledgment of the human condition. The second goal is the complete and final cessation of every form of suffering, leading to the attainment of *nirvana*. To attain nirvana, greed, hatred and delusion, which tie beings to the cycle of rebirth, must be eradicated (Rotem, 1996). The Four Noble Truths state that:

- Suffering is central to life: birth, ageing, sickness, death, parting, unfulfilled desires, decay, continual change and impermanence, all are suffering. "Even the 'I' or 'self' has no enduring quality, because in reality it is merely an error arising from false conceptualisation" (Rotem, 1996, p. 75).

- Suffering is caused by ignorance and desire (or craving: literally "thirst"): this includes the desire for sensual pleasure, for having more or less, for existence and for self-annihilation.

- Desire and suffering can be extinguished by following Buddhist discipline: by adhering to the disciplines followed by Buddha, the mind is purified and liberated. When the cause of suffering is understood the fires of greed, hatred and delusion can be "blown out". At this point the chain of craving and suffering is broken and the endless cycle of birth, death and rebirth is abandoned.

- The cessation of suffering through the elimination of desire is to be attained by following the Eightfold Noble Path: right speech, right action, right livelihood, right effort, right mindfulness, right concentration, right view and right thought (Dinh, 1998; Lounsbery, 1973; Rotem, 1996). "These eight factors affirm the three essential elements of Buddhist spiritual training: moral conduct, concentration and wisdom" (Rotem, 1996, p. 75).

Clinical Implications

Hong, whose case was described above, may not have sought help earlier for a number of reasons, but her Buddhist faith may have played an important role in her endurance of her suffering as she may have considered this to be her lot in life. As discussed in chapter 3, affective states that in the West would be labelled depressed may be considered normal in Buddhist cultures (Obeskeyere, 1985). Because the trials and suffering of everyday life are seen as a normal part of human existence, Buddhists are expected to meditate on these aspects of life and to come to terms with them to achieve the cessation of suffering (Obeskeyere, 1985). When a person becomes ill, help is often not sought in the early stages of the illness because "suffering, including physical pain, may be perceived as an integral part of one's life or as divine punishment for [desire or] unrighteous behaviour. It may be ignored, tolerated [uncomplainingly], or perceived as a symptom of disease" (Lien, n.d., p. 3; Luntz, 1998). A person's current suffering may be interpreted as retribution either for their own or their ancestors' unrighteous behaviour in previous incarnations and stoically accepted (Lien & Rice, 1994). Hong may, for example, have considered herself in some way responsible for her sister's death, perhaps because she was not present in Vietnam to prevent her death by drowning.

The tenets of the Buddhist belief system may lead to confusion when a clinician, who is doing a risk assessment, asks a Buddhist client such as Hong, whether she has had any thoughts about death, or of taking her life. Meditation may well involve contemplation of death, as death is the ultimate mark of the impermanence of life (Obeyeskere, 1985). An affirmative answer by the client may mean that she is meditating on death, not that she is contemplating suicide. On the other hand, an affirmative answer may be a cause for concern as Buddhism does not have strong sanctions against suicide (Kok, 1988). For Buddhists "afterlife is not an absolute one of heaven and hell, but just a prolongation of the cycles of reincarnation" (Kok, 1988, p. 238). In contrast, Western culture places a high value on life and the major role that mental health crisis services play in attempting to prevent suicide provides a measure of the value that is placed on the continuation of life (Zealberg, Hardesty & Tyson, 1998). To the major religions of Western culture, suicide is seen "as sinful and moral stigma is attached not only to the individual who commits suicide, but to all those related to him or her" (Young & Papadatou, 1997, p. 194). Attitudes to suicide, however, "vary from culture to culture since suicide may be regarded as sinful, as a criminal act, as a sign of weakness and madness, or ... as an honourable act serving a higher cause" (Young & Papadatou, 1997, p. 194).

To ensure that potential suicide plans are assessed as accurately as possible, the clinician should guard against the use of euphemisms regarding death and ask very specific, targeted questions regarding the client's attitude to suicide and about his plans to take his life. For example, the clinician should check the linguistic and cultural meaning of the word "suicide" with an interpreter or bilingual mental health professional.

The clinician assessing Hong faces some significant dilemmas. While the clinician may consider it important to find the means to alleviate her suffering, this may not be Hong's goal as she may see her suffering as part of life and as part of the pathway to enlightenment. The idea of suicide, on the other hand, may not seem as momentous to her as to the clinician, if she believes in the cycle of death and rebirth.

Confucianism

"... is a body of moral teachings that originated in China in the 6th century BC" (Chinnery, 1996a, p. 92). It is a philosophy of social and moral order, based on long current practices and institutions, in which status, age, obedience and virtue are venerated (Chinnery, 1996a; Lien, n.d.). Filial[1] piety and respect are emphasised and this regard is extended to include family ancestors, who are worshipped (Lien, n.d.).

> Families are rigidly hierarchical and age is venerated so that decisions relating to family wellbeing or individual needs are made by the eldest male in the family. The society is patriarchal, and women are expected to obey their fathers until marriage, their husband during marriage and their eldest son in widowhood (Luntz, n.d., p. 2).

The moral code of Confucianism prescribes a code of virtues, including altruism, courtesy, modesty, equity, urbanity, intelligence, honesty and moderation (Chinnery, 1996a; Minas & Evert, n.d.). The path of moderation suggests that "equilibrium is the ideal and anything too exaggerated is to be avoided. This has often been mistaken for passivity, placidity or even hypocrisy" (Minas & Evert, n.d., p. 34).

Clinical Implications

The clinical significance of the collectivist and high power distance values associated with Confucianism are explained in detail in chapter 2. One implication of Confucian teachings is that Western approaches to family intervention may need to be modified so that expectations regarding family hierarchy are observed. A clinician recounted how, in a family interview with a Chinese family, all the children (who were adolescents and adults) were very passive and would not contradict their father or speak up in front of him. If the family holds Confucian values, then the children would have been raised to accept their father's views on all matters and it would have been a breach of family rules and harmony to speak unless he invited them to do so. The clinician violated these family rules by inviting the children to express their views in front of their father, risking loss of face by the father. In this process the clinician's credibility may have been impaired.

Family dynamics of this kind might impair efforts to engage Hong's husband and parents-in-law in family work to discuss strategies for reducing her isolation and for improving her status in the family. If Hong and her husband's family hold Confucian values then she, and the family, would expect that she would show deference to the views of her father-in-law, her husband and her mother-in-law and would not feel free to express her own views in their presence.

Ancestor Worship and Spirit Possession

Ancestor worship existed before, but was popularised by Confucius. It is not a religious faith, but a philosophy that requires families to honour their dead

---

1 Filial: from *filius* son, and *filia* daughter. As in duty or sentiment due from a child to a parent (Brown, 1993).

(Minas & Evert, n.d.). Confucius taught that worship of ancestors could strengthen family ties and ensure family continuity (Chinnery, 1996a). The souls of ancestors are believed to be natural protectors of the family and to bring good fortune in business and other matters. Not to have descendants is a most unfilial act, as it signals disrespect to your parents and it means there will be no-one to keep an ancestral shrine and burn incense for you when you become an ancestor (Chinnery, 1996a). In addition to the burning of incense on anniversaries and other significant dates:

> ... the family might burn paper money to provide for the spirit's needs, and place offerings of food and drink in front of the altar. After reciting prayers, they would invite the ancestors to partake of the nourishment, although usually the living family will consume it in the end (Chinnery, 1996a, p. 107).

The help of ancestors will be sought if a family member is sick. Illness and misfortune are believed to be caused by the spirits of ancestors who have been displeased by a family member's actions (Minas & Evert, n.d.). Children are raised with the constant reminder that they must never bring shame on their ancestors (Dinh, 1998). An offended ancestral spirit can possess a person and such a spirit is believed to be capable of causing mental illness (Barrett, 1997; Kleinman, 1980; Luntz, 1998).

Clinical Implications

One implication of this belief is that the person with a mental illness (and/or their family) may be perceived as being to blame for the disorder, as it implies that they, or the family, have acted in a way that has offended their ancestors. These assumptions contribute to the stigma associated with mental illness in Asian cultures (Ng, 1997). Sue and Sue (1987), in the United States, observed that:

> ... although negative reactions to mental illness exist in the general public, the amount of stigma or shame associated with emotional difficulties is probably much greater among Asian American groups. Mental illness in a family member is considered a failure of the family system itself ... the failure or weakness of an individual is considered a disgrace to the family unit (p. 480).

A Hong Kong study found that only the most severely disturbed patients sought psychiatric help, but 20% did not present for more than a year after the onset of their disorder (Sue & Sue, 1987).

The spirit that possessed Hong was not an offended ancestral spirit but the ancestral spirit of her sister, who had died before her time and was wandering the world in search of a resting-place. Appropriate rituals, such as the burning of paper money and offerings, were required to help put her to rest and to provide for her in the afterlife. When Hong was made to drink water with ashes in it, prayers would have been written on the paper that was burnt to create the ashes.

For Hong, Ancestor Worship, Confucianism and Buddhism all contributed to her world-view and hence her conception of what was troubling her. For a clinician assessing Hong's mental state, each of these belief systems are relevant to understanding her disorder, and an understanding of the Asian world-view is important in making an accurate assessment.

Other important belief systems in Asian cultures include Taoism and supernatural beliefs.

Taoism

Taosim was founded in China by Lao Tzu in the 6th century BC (Chinnery, 1996b). Taoism, which has existed alongside Confucianism and Buddhism in China for centuries, is in many ways the antithesis of Confucianism. While Confucianism focuses on people as members of society, Taoism emphasises individual personal development and embraces the spirit world and the occult (Chinnery, 1996b). Tao, which means "the Way", is "the creative principle that orders the physical universe" (Chung-yuan, 1963; Dinh, 1998, p. 3). Taoism teaches that the individual can achieve happiness and contentment by seeking oneness with the Tao. This entails following the example of the natural world (Chinnery, 1996b). Non-action (*wu wei*) is the way to conform with nature. This does not mean doing nothing, but means not engaging in useless effort or in actions that conflict with nature, as such actions would only result in the opposite of what is intended. According to Taoism, individuals and the state will achieve much without external intervention. Life is perceived as being in a constant state of flux, but the Tao has a moderating influence over everything. Things that are pushed to extremes will be restored by the Tao to their previous state (Chinnery, 1996b).

In Chinese cosmology, the functioning of the universe, and everything in it, is based on the continuous interaction of the contrasting but complementary qualities of yin and yang (Lock, 1982). "It is the harmony of the spirits of yin and yang on which all harmony depends" (Chung-yuan, 1963, p. 138). Yin is the female element, representing negative energy, which produces darkness, coldness, wetness and emptiness. Yang, the male element, represents positive energy producing light, warmth, dryness and fullness (Dinh, 1998). When combined into one, yin and yang constitute ch'i, a vital life essence (see below) (Chung-yuan, 1963). People, as an extension of the cosmos, possess yin and yang qualities (*Am* and *Duong* in Vietnamese), and this applies to men and women alike (Sidel, 1975). The forces of yin and yang should be in balance for healthy physical and psychological functioning (Lock, 1982).

Illness may result from imbalance in the five interrelated organ systems and from blockage of the circulation of ch'i between the body parts (Kleinman, 1980; Lock, 1982). This may occur because the individual has deviated from "the Way" (Sidel, 1975). Taoism emphasises harmony through a blending with nature and avoidance of confrontation (Lien, n.d.; Luntz, 1998, Minas & Evert, n.d.). Harmony should govern one's relationships with others and with nature: if equilibrium is not maintained, then illness will result. The need to maintain balance between yin and yang is complemented by the requirement for balance between the "hot" and "cold" elements of the body. The terms hot and cold refer to elements of the body, and not to temperature. Imbalance in the hot and cold elements may also cause illness. An imbalance caused by an excess of hotness is treated by consuming foods that are classed as cold, while hot foods will be avoided (Dein & Lipsedge, 1998; Kleinman, 1980).

Ch'i. The Chinese concept of ch'i is similar to the Vietnamese *tinh khi* and refers to a vital essence of life, "that energizes thinking, judgement and emotions" (Barrett, 1997, p. 489). An illness concept widely reported throughout Asia is that of semen loss, which is thought to involve loss of ch'i and yang (the male principle). Semen loss is therefore viewed as a threat to health that may lead ultimately to death (Barrett, 1997, Kleinman, 1980), while "the keeping of one's seed … guarantees health and longevity" (Bhatia & Malik, 1991, pp. 691–692). Men presenting with semen-loss syndrome may complain of palpitations, dizziness, sweating, fatigue, weakness, anxiety, loss of appetite, guilt, and possibly, sexual dysfunction such as impotence or premature ejaculation (Barrett, 1997; Bhatia & Malik, 1991; Kleinman, 1980).

A Chinese case described by Kleinman (1980) provides an example of concerns over loss of ch'i:

> A Chinese American man, with a history of palpitations, dizziness, and sweating, refused to accept that tests demonstrated no abnormalities. He rejected the suggestion that he needed psychological treatment. He believed that he was sick with a "cold" disorder owing to loss of yang (male principle and therefore "hot") from too frequent intercourse with his new wife who was 14 years younger than him. He feared being unable to meet his wife's sexual needs and that his sickness would get worse because of the continuing reduction of yang through loss of semen. He had not disclosed this belief to his American doctors because he felt they might ridicule him (Kleinman, 1980).

Clinical Implications

Because Taoism teaches that balance, perfection and harmony will be gradually restored if nature is allowed to take its natural course without intervention, followers of Taoism may delay seeking help when mental health intervention might be required. (Dinh, 1998; Lock, 1982; Luntz, 1998). Western medicines may be rejected because they are believed to interfere with the natural harmony of the body (Luntz, 1998). Neuroleptics, for example, are seen as too "hot" and as having too much yang and hence are to be avoided, or "cold" foods are required to correct the imbalance (Dein & Lipsedge, 1998; Dinh, 1998).

> A Chinese patient needed hormone treatment for her condition, but was unwilling to take this because she considered hormone medication to be too hot. Her general practitioner investigated and found that by prescribing multivitamin tablets, which are considered to be cold, the patient felt that balance between the hot and cold elements could be achieved.

The next chapter illustrates how a clinician and a non-Western client were able to negotiate treatment with neuroleptics by determining how to correct imbalances in yin and yang caused by the medication.

Supernatural and Other Popular Beliefs

A range of supernatural and other types of beliefs are held in Asian cultures about the causes of mental illness. Psychosis may be attributed to the effects of a magic spell that has been cast upon the family member. The spell may be cast by an angry or jealous neighbour, some other malevolent person, a magician or a sorcerer who has used black magic (Dinh, 1998). However, psychosis may also be attributed to organic or hereditary factors (Sue & Sue, 1987).

According to popular belief in China, spirits and demons are thought to be responsible for the many ills that befall humanity. These spirits are to be found everywhere: in the trees, in caves, in the water, in the soil, in graves, and they throng in people's homes. If they enter and possess a person, they can cause mental illness (Sidel, 1975).

Minor mental illnesses may be attributed to lack of willpower, to thinking, worrying or studying too much and to weak nerves, as in neurasthenia (Dinh, 1998; Sue & Sue, 1987).

Hit by wind. Vulnerability to mental illness may be caused by being "hit by wind", a Vietnamese cultural belief. If the body is weak, then it is vulnerable to an attack of "wind", a common cause of physical illness throughout SouthEast Asia (Barrett, 1997). Wind is potentially "vicious" and harmful; therefore, people avoid exposure to drafts of air "for the wind could go through into your body and then be unable to get out, causing weakness, collapse and death" (Barrett, 1997, p. 489). Children are particularly vulnerable to wind. Once wind enters the body, it becomes vulnerable to harm by spirits. While wind cannot cause mental problems, it can make the body susceptible to penetration by spirits, which can affect the brain and lead to "craziness" (Barrett, 1997, p. 489). Spirits can cause symptoms such as speaking nonsense, behaving oddly and violent behaviour. If a child falls ill, incense may be burned and food offered to spirits to protect the child (Barrett, 1997).

Skin scratching is a common domestic remedy to "draw out" the wind and strengthen the nerves. It is done with either a coin or spoon, after ointment has been applied to the skin so that a weal is raised, but the skin is not broken (Barrett, 1997). Barrett (1997) describes a case of attack by wind:

> A Vietnamese man presented with the complaint that, during intercourse, he was caught by "a ball of wind" that moved around inside him causing a stomach-ache. This ball of wind came and went over several weeks, moving up and down his body, causing shortness of breath, tightness and numbness in his chest and fainting when it moved up into his head. He also complained of weakness, which was linked to semen loss. Psychosocial circumstances, including war and refugee experiences, current unemployment and the forthcoming birth of a new baby, were seen to be contributing factors. He was eventually diagnosed with adjustment disorder with panic attacks. He was considered recovered after a 6-month period, following a jointly negotiated treatment regime of a low to moderate dose of tricyclic antidepressants and coin scratching, which was administered by his brother-in-law (Barrett, 1997).

Explanatory Models in Asian Cultures

The complex synthesis of beliefs that contribute to the Asian world-view forms the background to the explanatory models of physical (and mental) illness in Asian cultures. A case example of the manner in which different aspects of these explanations may combine is offered by Kleinman (1980):

> An elderly woman with gastrointestinal problems is told by her shaman (see definition below) that she has an excess of internal hot energy or "fire" rising from her intestines that is blocking the circulation of air and blood. Rituals are performed to drive away "ghosts" and "bad things" that have caused the problem. These rituals involve writing movements above the woman's body with a brush and she is given paper charms and herbs to take with her (Kleinman, 1980).

Note that the explanatory model draws on both beliefs in spirit possession and the Taoist principle of balance between hot and cold elements.

Treatment of Spirit Possession

As already illustrated, a *shaman* (or *tang-ki* in Chinese) is likely to be consulted if someone is thought to be possessed. A shaman is a sacred folk healer, found in many cultures, who is "a 'master of spirits', who becomes voluntarily possessed by spirits in controlled circumstances and ... in a divinatory seance, both diagnoses and treats the misfortune (and illness) of the community" (Helman 1984, p. 219; Kleinman, 1980). In China the shaman, who practises in a temple, becomes possessed by his god in a trance and it is the god who heals, not the shaman (Kleinman, 1980). Shamans are often very poor, illiterate men or women who have been chosen by gods after having been cured by them of a life-threatening illness (Kleinman, 1980).

Taoist priests in Chinese cultures also conduct ceremonies to drive away or exorcise ghosts and evil spirits for problems that might be classed as medical or psychiatric from a Western perspective (Kleinman, 1980, Sidel, 1975). Geomancers[2] practice healing and divination, using, for example, the trigrams from the *I Ching* (Kleinman, 1980). Geomancers are secular healers who usually work outside temples, using divination to advise clients which type of treatment to undertake (Kleinman, 1980).

The belief systems underlying traditional Chinese and other Asian medicines result in a concern with the functioning of the person as an organic whole and in that sense differs from Western scientific medicine, which is concerned with the physical body, divided into its component parts (Kleinman, 1980). Because of this holistic conception of the person, Asian medicine takes an integrated approach to all illnesses, not distinguishing between body and mind (Fabrega, 1991).

Hong's Explanatory Model

With an understanding of some of the key aspects of Asian world-views, it is possible to speculate how Hong might have answered questions for eliciting her explanatory model:

Q. *What is your problem called?*

A. I am possessed by my dead sister's spirit.

Q. *What is the cause of your problem?*

A. My sister died before her time. I could not save her because I was not in Vietnam, and her spirit is searching for a resting place.

Q. *What does the spirit do to you, how does it work?*

A. It makes me and my son feel cold, as if we are dead. Sometimes my sister speaks through me, and sometimes she makes my head hurt so much that I have to try and run away and I can't bear to be stopped.

Q. *How serious is it?*

A. It is very serious, I think she wants to take my soul, and that of my son. [According to the family she has become violent, and her offerings to the ghost are excessive. The CAT Team considers her to be at risk because she has made threats with a knife and because she was contemplating suicide with her son.]

---

2 Geomancy is the achievement of harmony, physical and spiritual, between a person and their enivronment with regard to the placement of buildings or monuments. It is also divination by means of the figure made by a handful of earth thrown down at random, or figures or lines formed by a number of dots made at random (Macquarie Dictionary, 2001).

Q. *What treatment is needed?*

A. I need to make offerings to the ghosts, drink water with the ashes of burnt prayers and help my sister's spirit to find a resting place by getting help from a religious healer. [The family was relieved that Hong received professional treatment that alleviated her symptoms. Following Hong's discharge from the inpatient unit, the CAT Team followed her up for some time, linking her with English classes and a Vietnamese women's group.]

Q. *What will the outcome be?*

A. If my sister's spirit can find rest, then she will no longer possess me. [The CAT Team reported that Hong showed no further evidence of psychosis and formed several friendships in the women's group. Hong's family suggested to her that in future it would not be a good idea to tell Western people about her beliefs in spirits if she did not want to be put into hospital against her will again.]

This last piece of advice by Hong's family illustrates that non-Western clients may not always be willing to disclose their beliefs in the supernatural as they fear that their beliefs may be misinterpreted or ridiculed (Kleinman, 1980). This issue is addressed further in the next chapter on Negotiating Explanatory Models.

The Place of Religion in Western and non-Western Societies

Many of the beliefs we have discussed have their base in religion. For many people, particularly in non-Western cultures:

> *Religion is not just an important part of their lives but rather the central focus around which everything else revolves.* Religion provides an overarching framework in which they conceptualise their world. It structures everyday experiences and plays an important role in articulating their distress, providing an explanation of suffering and misfortune ... (Dein & Lipsedge, 1998, p. 145; emphasis added).

Wessells illustrates the impact of spiritual beliefs in war-torn regions of Africa:

> Throughout Bantu areas of Africa, spirituality is at the centre of life and some of the most significant effects of war ... are spiritually based. If a boy's mother were killed in an attack and he fled the village without burying her, this could be a great source of stress for him. In failing to conduct the appropriate burial ritual, the boy is likely to believe that his mother's spirit is unavenged, causing problems for him and those with whom he is in contact. Healing may require the conduct of a culturally relevant ritual of burial or of purification to restore spiritual harmony (Wessells, 1997, p. 14).

In Western society, however, Kleinman (1988) argues that spiritual beliefs have lost their significance:

> The rationalising powers of modern secular ... society have either created or intensified a metaself — a critical observer who watches and comments on experience. The self is alienated from unreflected, unmediated experience. By internalising a critical observer, the self is rendered inaccessible to possession by gods or ghosts; it cannot faint from fright or become paralysed by humiliation; it loses the literalness of bodily metaphors of the most intimate personal distress, accepting in their place a psychological metalanguage that has the appearance of immediacy but in fact distances felt experience; and the self becomes vulnerable to forms of pathology (like borderline and narcissistic personality disorders) that appear culture-bound to the West (Kleinman, 1988, p. 50).

Gaines (1982) argues that two major cultural traditions can be distinguished in the Western world-view. The Northern European Culture Area "is home to the world view which Weber (1963) referred to as 'disenchanted'" and was influenced by the Protestant Reformation from which arose "a practical, empiricist, non-magical approach to the social and natural worlds" (Gaines, 1982, p. 179). This is distinguished from the enchanted world view of the Mediterranean Culture Area where illnesses are understood as having either natural or supernatural causes, such as fate, spirits or devils. Gaines (1982) argues that biomedicine and psychiatry are heir to the former tradition. With the search for a biological source for mental disorder, the need to understand clients in their psychosocial and cultural context tends to be de-emphasised and the important function of the "healing nexus", created by the meaningful acts of the professional healer, may be overlooked (Gaines, 1982, p. 176).

While religion and spirituality may be among the most important aspects of human experience, the mental health sector has tended to ignore clients' religious or spiritual views, or else pathologised them as hallucinatory or delusional symptoms (Lukoff, Lu & Turner, 1995). Lack of familiarity with other cultures' belief systems increases the risk of misdiagnosing another's religious ideas, but with the framework we have provided a clinician can learn from the client and family what beliefs they hold. Clinical judgement is then required to differentiate culturally accepted beliefs from mental illness.

Differentiating Mental Illness from Culturally Sanctioned Beliefs

The "bizarre" experiences reported by Hong, Samuel and Danny are considered bizarre from a Western perspective because they are outside the normative experiences of Western cultures. Clinicians, and, for that matter, the lay population, "know" that people cannot be possessed by spirits, they cannot be affected by spells, and they cannot hear voices in the absence of auditory stimuli. This is cultural knowledge that is taken for granted (Kleinman, 1980). But this taken-for-granted normative reality is challenged when a person of a non-Western background reports experiences that appear to be sanctioned within that person's culture. The cultural relativity of normative boundaries becomes apparent in such a context.

Part of the clinician's task then is to determine to what extent the non-Western client's experiences fall within normative boundaries for that culture (Lefley et al., 1998; Kleinman, 1996). Eliciting the client's (and the family's) explanatory model and gaining an understanding of the underlying belief system are crucial steps in making these normative judgements. This process is discussed in detail in the next chapter; however, broad criteria for differentiating between psychotic behaviour and spiritual behaviours are required to guide such an interview.

A number of authors have attempted to provide such distinguishing criteria, but some are too specific to a particular belief system and some include dubious criteria (Helman, 1984; Lefley et al., 1998; Westermeyer, 1987). Sharp (1994), in writing about spirit possession in Madagascar, makes the generally useful point that spirit possession and madness represent opposite ends of a continuum, although their causation, symptoms and treatment overlap. It is the severity of symptoms that distinguish between madness and possession. This was well illustrated by the case of Hong, whose offerings to the spirits far exceeded normal practices. Sharp (1994) argues that "madness" is "defined very broadly by deviant forms of behaviour" where the "breaking of social norms is of major significance" (Sharp, 1994, p. 528). This point is included as the first and a crucial criterion in our set of criteria. Whether norms have been broken is usually best established by asking the family or the cultural reference group. Other criteria drawn from the literature and from our own clinical experience suggest that the following questions should be asked and observations made in distinguishing culturally sanctioned beliefs from delusions:

- Do the beliefs worry the client's family or cultural reference group?
- Has there been a deterioration in functioning?
- Are the beliefs associated with risk behaviour?

Consider the client's beliefs in the context of the overall assessment of the client's mental state: are there other aspects of the client's functioning that are a matter of concern (e.g., deterioration in self-care)? If so, then unusual spiritual beliefs should be seen in this context.

The Creation of Clinical Reality: Transformation of the Client's Suffering

When the individual decides they have an illness and moves out of the popular and into the expert sector of the health care system, whether traditional or professional, their sick role is redefined (Good & Good, 1982; Kleinman, 1980). Each type of clinical practice creates a "clinical reality", with beliefs about and attitudes to sickness, normative expectations regarding the behaviours of a sick person, expectations concerning treatment adherence and expectations regarding responses by the family and by the practitioner to the sick person (Kleinman, 1980). The effect of these implicit expectations in the different health care sectors is that the person's everyday experience of suffering is *transformed* into the illness categories of traditional healers or the biomedical model (Kleinman & Kleinman, 1991). In each setting the client's "illness is perceived, labelled and interpreted, and a special form of care is applied. Each arena has entrance and exit roles and rules" (Kleinman, 1980, p. 52). The sick person must translate the semantic meanings of one sector's language to another as he or she moves from one health care system to another. An individual's conceptualisation of their disorder will not only determine the type of help sought, but is also likely to influence the symptoms reported and adherence to treatment (Angel & Thoits, 1987).

Because of the different languages of each health care sector, the patient and clinician may disagree about the nature of the disorder (Kleinman, 1980). The Chinese patient who believed his palpitations and dizziness were due to hot/cold imbalances caused by excessive semen loss may not share a Western mental health professional's view that he is suffering from an anxiety disorder (i.e., a mental disorder). However, the professional sector's definition of illness and concomitant treatment are likely to prevail over popular definitions because the professional sector has greater legitimate power through its institutionalised role (Kleinman, 1980). Nevertheless, the Chinese patient can sidestep the professional sector by turning to a shaman in the traditional sector, where his interpretation of his illness experience *is* more likely to be shared.

To avoid losing clients in the mental health sector through unacknowledged discrepancies in explanatory models, the mental health professional needs the tools and skills to identify and negotiate these differences to achieve a shared understanding. The process of negotiation is described in a transcript of a crosscultural clinical interview in the next chapter, followed by a cultural formulation of the case.

Conclusion

In this chapter we have examined how explanatory models arise in the context of a belief system or world-view. As part of our crosscultural framework for understanding a client's perception of their problem we have also considered the health care systems associated with the various belief systems and the way that cultures differ in defining illness. To illustrate we looked at a range of crosscultural beliefs relating to illness, in particular, the belief systems of the evil eye and various Asian beliefs (termed for our purposes, "Asian world-views"). This has by no means been a totally comprehensive account of different belief systems as they relate to illness, and even within one culture, no two clients will hold identical beliefs; however, we hope to have provided clinicians with a model to follow in eliciting the belief systems of clients from other cultures.

Negotiating Explanatory Models

Discrepancies Between Explanatory Models

On entering the mental health system, the explanatory model of the non-Western client is transformed into the biomedical explanatory model of the mental health practitioner, as explained in chapter 6. As part of the transformation the client is expected to comprehend the benefit of and comply with the treatment that is consonant with the biomedical model. If, however, the treatment or intervention does not match with the beliefs, cultural lifestyle and norms of the patient, he or she may not cooperate with treatment, or terminate treatment prematurely (Sue & Zane, 1987). For example, if a 28-year-old, single Greek man is told that, as part of his treatment for a serious mental illness, he should learn independent living skills (such as cooking and shopping) he may consider this to be inconsistent with the normative expectations associated with the male sex role in his culture. Similarly, if a Lebanese family is told that their young daughter is to be admitted to a mixed sex inpatient unit for her safety, it is possible that the family may not cooperate because this may be seen to compromise her honour.

The process by which discrepancies in understanding can be negotiated will be described in this chapter, followed by a transcript of a clinical interview illustrating one approach to negotiation.

The aims of eliciting explanatory models and negotiating differences are:

- to gain as full as possible an understanding of the client's illness

- to work as far as possible within the client's framework

- to avoid the client gaining the impression that the clinician regards their explanatory model as ridiculous or ignorant

- to avoid imposing on the client a view of the illness that does not make sense to them.

The clinician's role in negotiating explanatory models can be summarised as:

- eliciting the client's explanatory model

- communicating the mental health model in plain language

- showing respect for the client's framework and acknowledging any significant discrepancies in conceptualisation

- negotiating by looking for common ideas and finding common ground

- finding a way to accommodate Western treatment to the client's framework (e.g., working with a herbalist)

- accommodating the patient's treatment expectations, rather than adopting the client's framework.

Eliciting the Client's Explanatory Model

Before discrepancies in explanatory models can be identified, the clinician first needs to elicit the patient's explanatory model, with an awareness that such models may not be "fully articulated, may be less abstract [than the medical model], may be inconsistent and even self-contradictory, and may be based on erroneous evaluation of evidence" (Kleinman et al., 1978, p. 256). Elicitation may involve asking key questions, which were discussed in chapter 5, about their explanatory model. Prior to asking these questions, the clinician needs to explain to the client that they need to obtain a good understanding of how the client understands the problem so that the most effective treatment can be agreed upon.

Clients may be reluctant to disclose their explanatory models to clinicians for fear of ridicule. To deal with this the clinician will need to be warm, empathic and persistent to show patients that they are genuinely interested and that their ideas are important in formulating optimal treatment plans (Kleinman, 1982; Kleinman et al., 1978). Because explanatory models may be only partly conscious, involving implicit knowledge, the client may only gradually be able to verbalise their explanatory model (Kleinman, 1980; Leventhal et al., 1980). Because it is implicit, it may be difficult for the clinician to see that the explanatory model does function, at any one time, as an organised system that helps the client to explain their experience (Leventhal et al., 1980). Patients may conceal their non-compliance with treatment because they fear confrontation between their personal theories of illness and those of the clinician. They may be reluctant to challenge the clinician's authority for fear of loss of support or derision (Leventhal et al., 1980).

The clinician also needs to be aware that a client's explanatory model may not be static. It may contain internal contradictions and may shift when the client becomes unwell. At this time the client may revert to their parents' explanatory model, although this may have been rejected in the past, as illustrated by the case of Danny in the previous chapter. This may occur with both Western and non-Western clients. For example, an Australian-born client who is secular in their beliefs when well, may become religious when unwell, and then revert to a secular world-view when they recover. Similarly an acculturated non-Western client may move from a Western explanatory model while well, to an explanatory model from their culture of origin when unwell. The client may retain this belief upon recovery, or resume belief in a Western explanatory model, or hold aspects of both cultures' explanatory models side by side. In a typical pathway to care, those suffering from an illness will change their explanatory model if the treatments attempted prove unsuccessful, relative to their expectations.

It is also important to elicit the explanatory models held by the more powerful members of the client's family, to identify potential conflicts between the explanatory models held by the clinician, by the client's family and by the client (Kleinman et al., 1978). Often, different members of a family may hold different models of illness. Occasionally this may lead to conflict and disagreement about the need for treatment and about the type of treatments that will be accepted. Disagreement about the severity, likely course, outcome and social consequences of the illness may affect the motivation to seek help. Disagreements about the cause and meaning of an illness may influence what therapeutic options are adopted. The case of Anh later in this chapter illustrates that when the treatment proposed is not consistent with the explanatory model of a key family member, the client may be discouraged from cooperating with treatment.

Communicating the Mental Health Model in Plain Language

The mental health clinician should be able formulate and communicate their explanatory model of mental illness in clear language that the client can understand. The formulation should address the seven key concerns of name, cause, reason for timing of onset, pathology, severity, course and outcome, and treatment (Kleinman et al., 1978). Our experience has been, when training clinicians, that few felt confident that they could convey the mental health model in clear, concise terms — an issue that seemed to be related to the lack of certainty regarding the causes of mental illness. Often, mental disorders are described, rather than explained. Thus, clinicians may provide the name of the disorder (which is often incomprehensible to the client and family), its symptomatology and the prescribed treatment (Collins et al., 2002). More comprehensive explanations may make reference to factors such as family heredity, neurochemical imbalances, vulnerability, triggering or stress factors. These explanations, however, are rife with biomedical assumptions that would be unfamiliar to many non-Western clients. Kleinman et al. (1978) suggest that:

> ... part of systematic clinical practice should be an attempt to articulate the doctor's model in simple and direct terms for each of the ... major issues of clinical concern. Students should be taught how to communicate the medical model to patients (p. 257).

A clinician may want to communicate a social work or psychological model, rather than a medical model. Whatever the model, developing a clear explanatory model can be confronting to clinicians as they endeavour to articulate their framework of practice in lay language. While it is the task of the clinician to communicate their illness model as simply as possible, it is *not* their task to convince the client that this model is correct and the client's model is mistaken.

The clinician's lay explanatory model should be credible and should incorporate the various aspects of the client's illness experience (Kleinman, 1982). Fitzpatrick (1984) found that patients presenting with physical symptoms were likely to accept a medical practitioner's explanations:

> Only when two conditions were met: if they were provided with adequate information, allowing them to appreciate the significance of their symptoms; and if the affective meaning of their symptoms was elicited by their doctor, so that the patient felt that the doctor had understood his or her perspective on the symptoms (Fitzpatrick, 1984, p. 28).

Factors contributing to credibility will be discussed in the next section.

Angel and Thoits (1987) suggest that contact with mental health professionals' explanatory models tends to influence popular lay explanations of illness. "Professional labelling and evaluation is 'fed back' into the cultural system when the individual communicates the outcome to others" (p. 483). They argue that during the process of acculturation a gradient of explanatory models exists in migrant communities, from the more traditional to the more scientifically oriented. The clinical implication is that a client's explanatory model may change from a traditional to a more biomedical explanatory model over the course of their treatment.

Acknowledging and Showing Respect for the Client's Framework and any Significant Discrepancies in Conceptualisation

Once the client's explanatory model has been respectfully acknowledged and the clinician's explanatory model has been made explicit, discrepancies between the explanatory models can be identified. The clinician should make explicit comparisons between the models, pointing out the discrepancies, but always maintaining respect for the client's conceptualisation. The client should be encouraged to ask questions about the clinician's model and the discrepancies, which can inform the clinician about aspects of the model that need to be clarified for the client. These questions may also help to reveal central concerns for the client (Kleinman et al., 1978).

Negotiating by Looking for Common Ideas and Finding Common Ground

If treatment and intervention are to be successful, conflicts between models need to be reduced by a process of negotiation to reach a mutually acceptable explanatory model. This negotiated model will help to justify the treatment approach and gain the patient's cooperation. As an important aspect of negotiating a shared model the clinician should look for ideas that are common to, or similar, in the two explanatory models. If common ground can be found it forms a strong basis for negotiation (G. Coffey, personal communication, November, 1998). This may involve obtaining the client's agreement that the family thinks certain of the client's behaviours are outside normative limits and require treatment (see the case of Anh), or it may mean that the client has adopted aspects of the clinician's model. At this stage the clinician "actively negotiates with the patient [as a therapeutic ally,] about treatment and expected outcomes" (Kleinman et al., 1978, p. 256). Negotiation should not overlook the family's explanatory model, particularly if this is discrepant with the client's model. As previously stated, family support is vital if a negotiated treatment is to be successful with a client from a collectivist culture. This will also be demonstrated in the case study of Anh.

Accommodating Western Treatment to the Client's Framework

As part of the negotiation process the clinician may agree to provide treatment in collaboration with a traditional healer such as a herbalist or shaman, or a religious leader. Alternatively, for example, the client may wish to counter the "hot" effects of psychotropic medication with "cold" foods or remedies. As long as the traditional treatment does not counteract the clinical treatment, there is no reason why clients should be discouraged from these courses of action. On the contrary, they should be supported (Walter & Rey, 1999).

Accommodating the Client's Treatment Expectations Rather than Adopting the Client's Framework

Clinicians may feel that they will make better progress in negotiating explanatory models if they adopt the client's explanatory model; for example, agreeing with the client that they are possessed by an angry spirit. If the clinician does not believe this then it is dishonest to pretend to do so. This may also impair the clinician's credibility, as the client is unlikely to accept that the clinician also subscribes to the client's belief system.

Credibility is an important ingredient in successful negotiation of shared explanatory models. Other ingredients are respect and the provision of benefit.

Factors Contributing to Successful Negotiation: Respect, Credibility and Provision of Benefit

Respect

We have already mentioned the importance of showing respect when asking a client to explain their conceptualisation of their illness. Wessels (1997), who has worked with trauma victims in Angola and Sierra Leone, suggests that people from those cultures may view their own traditional practices and views as backward and may be reluctant to talk about them with clinicians. Without intending to, it is easy to subtly marginalise the individual's cultural knowledge and impose a Western clinical view. Wessells (1997) suggests that a relationship of mutual respect is best established by telling a person that you want to learn from them and with them, enabling a blending of cultures and approaches. Respectful discussion may rekindle commitment to cultural traditions that may have been disrupted by resettlement (Wessells, 1997).

Credibility

Sue and Zane (1987) explored the issue of credibility in their work with Asian clients. They argue that "credibility" and "giving" are vital factors in negotiating treatment with non-Western clients. A clinician achieves credibility when they are perceived as a trustworthy and effective helper. Sue and Zane maintain that there are improved therapeutic outcomes for clients if they believe in the therapist and the methods they employ. Credibility, they suggest, is the product of two factors: ascribed status and achieved status.

Ascribed status. Is the position or role that is assigned to an individual by others (Sue & Zane, 1987). The individual occupying the role is not required to first prove that they are deserving of status. Certain roles attract ascribed status, including monarchs and, in most cultures, doctors. Culture strongly influences a person's role in the social hierarchy. In traditional Asian cultures the aged tend to have ascribed status and, therefore, can exert authority over the young. Similarly, men exert authority over women and the learned over the less educated (Sue & Zane, 1987; see also chapter 2). But status and, therefore, credibility can be achieved.

Achieved status. May be attained through clinical skills. Non-Western clients may recognise and accord status to nurses and doctors, but they may not be familiar with roles such as counsellors, occupational therapists, psychologists and social workers. As a result, clinicians filling the allied health roles may initially lack credibility with non-Western clients as they do not have an ascribed status. However, status, and thus credibility, can be achieved through the therapeutic actions of the clinician, enabling the client to develop confidence, hope and trust (Sue & Zane, 1987).

Discrepancies in credibility would occur if, for example, the clinician was a young woman known to have a high level of expertise (Sue & Zane, 1987).

In this case the age and gender of the therapist would be associated with low ascribed status, but her expertise may compensate allowing her to achieve status and, therefore, credibility (Sue & Zane, 1987).

Sue and Zane (1987) suggest that three factors can impair credibility:

1. If the clinician conceptualises the client's problems in a manner that is incongruent with the client's belief system.

2. If the clinician proposes means of resolving the problem that require the client to act in a culturally unacceptable or incompatible manner.

3. If the clinician's and client's treatment goals are discrepant.

Although, medical practitioners tend to have high ascribed status and credibility in most cultures, their credibility would diminish if, for example, they failed to conceptualise a client's problem in terms that were consistent with the client's conceptualisation. Knowledge of the cultural values of an ethnic group can facilitate a clinician's analysis of existing and potential credibility issues in a clinical transaction (Sue & Zane, 1987).

Giving: Provision of Benefit

"Giving" is the client's perception that something was received from the clinical encounter (Sue & Zane, 1987). While it is important for a shared explanatory model to be negotiated between the clinician and client, the negotiated understanding needs to be given credibility by providing the client with a direct benefit from treatment (Kleinman, 1980; Sue & Zane, 1987). Sue and Zane (1987) call this benefit a "gift", "because gift giving is a ritual that is frequently a part of interpersonal relationships among Asians" (p. 42). The very act of seeking to understand the client's illness model may be viewed as a form of giving, but other kinds of gifts are required to demonstrate that the client's problems are able to be treated. Treatment benefits should be provided early in the clinical encounter (preferably during the first clinical transaction). Examples of gifts include:

• Alleviating or reducing negative emotional states such as depression and anxiety.

• Providing cognitive clarity for a client in a state of crisis and confusion.

• Providing medication to help control out-of-control emotional or cognitive states.

• "Normalising" the client's feelings, thoughts and experiences by assuring them that many people have similar experiences in similar situations (while not minimising the individual's unique experience) (Sue & Zane, 1987).

• Providing reassurance, hope, coping skills and goal setting (Sue & Zane, 1987).

Providing these benefits to the client can also benefit anxious families.

The case of Hong, presented in the section on Asian world-views in the previous chapter, provides a useful example of the role of credibility and gift giving. Hong said she was possessed by the spirit of her dead sister and spoke as the spirit of her sister. The treating medical officer on the crisis team effectively engaged Hong by asking the sister's spirit for permission to treat the client. Analysis of credibility and gift giving suggests that if the client has not previously encountered a crisis team, then these teams would have low ascribed status and therefore lack credibility with the client because they are an unfamiliar service. On the other hand, the crisis team may have benefited from the ascribed status of the medical practitioner who was present as a member of the team. Acknowledgement by the clinician of the possessing spirit and its power may be perceived as a gift, with the promise of relief from the distress caused by the spirit. This process may have contributed to the achieved status of the crisis team, which increased its credibility in the eyes of the client. We will now examine an example of the process of negotiation by analysing material emerging from a series of clinical interviews. This is followed by a cultural formulation of the case.

A Clinical Session Illustrating Negotiation Strategies

Background Information on Anh

Anh is a single, Vietnamese woman aged 30, who came to Australia in 1994, at the age of 24, to marry a Vietnamese man whom she had met in Vietnam. He had left the country 2 years earlier and sponsored her move to Australia. Anh, who is the third in a family of five children, left behind three of her siblings and her mother. Her father died in a re-education camp. When she arrived in Australia she lived with her sister (a student), initially on a temporary basis, while her fiancé worked to buy a house. For a time she worked in a small Vietnamese video shop, but started having arguments with people in the adjoining shop and was sacked by her employer.

Six months after arriving in Australia, Anh was diagnosed with schizophrenia and her fiancé rejected her. Shortly afterwards he married another Vietnamese woman and refused to have anything to do with Anh, although Anh pleaded with him to keep his promise to marry her. She visited him several times at his work until his employer forbade her to enter the workplace. She then found out whom he had married and began to harass the wife on the phone and at home, accusing her of stealing her husband. The couple changed their phone number to a silent number and were eventually obliged to take out an intervention order forbidding Anh to enter their street, or to come within 200 metres of them.

This all happened some 3–4 years ago, but Anh remains preoccupied with her former fiancé, hallucinating his voice and considering it her fate to marry him. Anh is a practising Buddhist. She continues to live with her sister who has since married and has two young children. Her sister works at a council as a child support worker and is quite supportive of Anh, but gets angry with her when she becomes unwell and does not carry out her allocated domestic duties. Two months ago her sister's family moved to a different suburb and Anh's management has been taken over by another mental health service. The referring mental health service had diagnosed Anh as having schizophrenia and placed her on a compulsory community treatment order because she was non-compliant with medication.

This background information has been elicited in the initial assessment interviews and in subsequent sessions.[1] The transcript of interview that follows is composed of extracts from a session that occurred some two months after the initial assessment interview, after which time Anh had developed some trust in her clinician. Tom West is the treating clinician, a clinical psychologist with extensive experience in crosscultural clinical work. Tom, in the process of reviewing Anh's progress, has developed a therapeutic relationship with Anh and they meet once a week. As Anh speaks English at a low-to-moderate level of proficiency, the session is being conducted with a Vietnamese interpreter who is experienced in working in mental health settings, to ensure accurate two-way communication. Tom previously established that Anh speaks Vietnamese[2] and that she would prefer a female interpreter. Anh trusts the interpreter because she has met her at the previous mental health service she attended.

An important aspect of this case is that cultural beliefs and psychotic symptoms are intertwined in a way that is difficult to disentangle. Comments accompany the interview transcript to illustrate how the separate strands of culturally normative beliefs and psychosis are teased out. In addition, the clinician uses his versions of the explanatory model questions to elicit Anh's understanding of her problem, negotiates discrepancies in their respective explanatory models and then employs negotiation strategies to obtain cooperation with treatment. Readers are encouraged to watch for these elements as they occur in the interview and to judge how effective the various strategies are. In particular, consider how well the Western explanatory model of mental illness is conveyed and what approach you might use.

Note that this transcript represents extracts from a series of interviews that highlight cultural features. In reality this material might take several interviews to elicit and the discussion is likely to be interspersed with other topics not specifically related to culture.

---

1 To ensure anonymity the background to this case is a compilation of the background to several actual cases. The interview is an edited transcription of a role-played interview by two clinicians, Guy Coffey and Thuy Dinh.

2 Country of origin does not necessarily correlate with language spoken (i.e., there are a number of ethnic Chinese in Vietnam who speak a Chinese language, not Vietnamese).

We suggest that the reader first read the interview transcript in the left-hand column straight through, disregarding the commentary in the right-hand column. This will enable the reader to obtain a coherent sense of the interview, and to make some preliminary personal judgements about the nature of the cultural issues that arise, and the interview technique. After this, the reader may return to compare their own conclusions with those in the commentary on the interview.

Extracts from a Clinical Interview

Interview Transcript   Commentary

Tom: And how is it going in the household, are you happy living with Tuyet [Anh's sister]?

> Tom opens up the discussion on potential household difficulties.

Anh: No.

Tom: What kind of problems are there?

Anh: Um, a ghost.

Tom: A ghost. What do you mean by that?

> Anh provides a reply that is pregnant with diagnostic possibilities, but first Tom needs to examine the meaning Anh gives to the word "ghost".

Anh: There is a ghost in our house.

Tom: So tell me about that Anh; how do you know that there is a ghost there?

> Tom does not immediately assume Anh is suffering from hallucinations or delusions but respectfully asks questions to explore the experiential basis of Anh's belief that there is a ghost in the house. Is it something someone told her? Is it based on hallucinatory experiences? Or is it a culturally normative experience? In this process he is beginning to elicit the explanatory model around her current concerns.

Anh: Ghosts are everywhere; they're everywhere! They're in Vietnam; they're here. Ghosts are everywhere, I know.

> Anh's answer carries a strong sense of conviction that ghosts are present in both countries. This may reflect Anh's fear of ghosts or an attempt to be convincing. Tom will shortly attempt to verify whether this is a culturally accepted belief.

Tom: Have you seen or heard the ghost?

> Tom begins to assess how the ghost is experi-
> enced and what kind of "evidence" Anh uses to
> support her belief. Her answers may provide a
> context for assessing whether or not she is experi-
> encing hallucinations. Here Tom asks directly if
> she has had any relevant sensory experiences that
> would indicate she has personally "encountered"
> the ghost.

Anh: I hear noises. At night.

Tom: What kind of noises do you hear?

Anh: I've heard walking steps at night; the ghost moves things around and I have heard people crying.

Tom: And you believe that is due to a ghost in the house?

Anh: Yes.

Tom: So how does it affect you, having a ghost in the house?

> Up to this point Anh's answers have provided
> Tom with evidence that, from the perspective of a
> Western explanatory model, suggests that Anh's
> illness may involve auditory hallucinations. By
> attributing these experiences to ghosts, Anh has
> implicitly answered Kleinman's explanatory model
> question, "What has caused your problem?". Now
> Tom asks the equivalent of the explanatory model
> question, "What does this sickness do to you?"

Anh: I'm scared.

Tom: Anh, do you know why this is happening? Why is there a ghost in the house?

> Tom returns to exploration of the social, personal
> and historical context of the identified cause. Is
> there a precipitating circumstance? This is akin to
> asking Kleinman's key question, "Why do you
> think it started when it did?". This may help in
> distinguishing culturally normative beliefs from
> symptoms of illness.

Anh: When my grandmother died she came back to talk to us.

> Anh volunteers information about the social
> context in which ghosts appear in her culture and,
> incidentally, gives her own cultural definition of
> what ghosts are.

Tom: When was that?

Anh: That was a long time ago. She came back and talked to us, to my mum; everybody knew that she was coming. She talked to us a lot.

> Anh acknowledges that events surrounding
> her grandmother occurred in the past. The
> grandmother's "return" is presented as a shared

family experience and, emotionally, the "visit" does not have the same tone as the current "ghost" experiences. Anh's claim that others also heard her grandmother's voice suggests that this may have been a culturally acceptable experience.

Tom: So, on that occasion you knew why the ghost came to you. It was associated with your grandmother.

Tom implicitly acknowledges the difference between the culturally normative experience of the grandmother's ghost and the current ghost. This helps Anh to return to the initial conversation from which she may have strayed due to a loosening of associations. Tom is aware that in some cultures when a loved relative has died, family members may hear the deceased person's voice, may see them in dreams, when falling asleep or when waking up. But it is not clear whether this is what is troubling Anh now.

Anh: But this is not my grandmother, my grandmother is in Vietnam. This is the ghost of the dead bodies buried under the house.

Anh acknowledges that the ghost that is presently disturbing her is not that of a loved deceased relative. Is her present experience of the ghost culturally normative?

Tom: Have you discussed this with Tuyet at all?

To test this, Tom asks whether the sister has experienced the ghost as in the case of the grandmother's ghost, possibly normalising Anh's experience. Or, is this a private experience that her own sister regards as abnormal? Has Anh attempted to resolve the problem of the ghost using her social network (the popular sector of the healthcare system)? Would this approach be a culturally appropriate "treatment?"

Anh: She knows, she knows that ghosts are everywhere. She believes it. She hears the noise as well.

Tom: What is her opinion about the ghost?

Anh: She said, ummm, that spirits come back — people die and their spirit comes back.

Tom persists and Anh returns an uncertain answer that does not allay Tom's suspicion that the ghost is experienced by her alone. It would appear that Tuyet has tried to conceptualise Anh's experience as normal, although it is not certain that she, herself, has heard this ghost.

Tom: And Anh, why do you think the spirit is coming to you?

> Tom returns to the issue of the "cause behind the cause" (i.e., the social context of her ghost experience), at the same time exploring whether there are grandiose/paranoid aspects to Anh's belief. Does she believe she is special and that she has been singled out by the ghost for a reason?

Anh: The spirit comes to everybody. The spirit comes to Tuyet too.

> Together with the story of her grandmother, Anh appears very keen to communicate that her experience is normal.

Tom: Was it your experience in Vietnam Anh, that spirits came to people there?

Anh: Yes.

Tom: So did you hear people talking about this happening to them in Vietnam?

> By asking about social and family attitudes to ghosts, Tom is not only establishing the extent to which they are culturally accepted phenomenon, but also he is according significance to the primary role the family plays in collectivist cultures in influencing individual opinions and values.

Anh: Oh yes, a lot.

Tom: Including in your own family?

Anh: Yes, my mum.

> At this point it seems that both Anh and her family believe in ghosts. Tom will, however, talk to the family.

Tom: And what was their opinion about why spirits came at particular times?

> For now Tom seeks additional information about the ghost, which communicates to Anh both that he is willing to explore her story and also that he will not ridicule her ideas.

Anh: Sometimes they are hungry, they want food, sometimes they want to scare you.

Tom: And is there anything you or Tuyet have done about the ghost? Is there anything you can do to make it affect you less?

> While acknowledging that the ghost experience is shared with her sister, and while acceding to Anh's insistence that her experience is within normal limits, Tom directly asks his own version of Kleinman's question "What treatment do you think you should receive?"

Anh: We go to the Buddhist temple and ask the monk to come to the house and bless it with holy water and we have to make an offering of food every month to the ghost so that it won't cause any trouble.

> Notably Tom has not questioned whether the sister has experienced the ghost, despite his doubts. Tom's patience is rewarded when he learns that both sisters perform ritual offerings to ward off danger from the ghost.

Tom: Has that been effective? Has that made the ghost's presence affect you less?

> Tom enquires about the effectiveness of cultural solutions. Perhaps if the cultural strategy has not been effective Anh may be motivated to receive an alternative. This creates an opportunity for negotiation and for the offering of a gift or benefit.

Anh: No. Sometimes. Not all the time, sometimes. I heard the ghost again yesterday.

Tom: And you are still feeling quite frightened by the ghost. All right, Anh, tell me a bit about how you are living your day-to-day life? When Tuyet was with us at the last appointment, do you recall she said that you were spending most of the day in your room and that you seemed very frightened? Why are you doing that?

> Tom acknowledges the distress and fear that Anh is experiencing and will return to address this issue below. For now he maintains a broad perspective, exploring the psychosocial context in which the situation has developed. He focuses particularly on family reports that are suggestive of withdrawal and fearful or paranoid behaviour. As this appears to be another sign of Anh's sickness Tom asks about the "cause" behind this behaviour.

Anh: People are really bad. They say bad things about me.

> Somewhat surprisingly Anh moves off the topic of ghosts and now focuses on interpersonal relationships (although the emotional tone of persecution persists into the new theme).

Tom: Do you hear them saying these things to you even when you are in your bedroom alone?

> Tom is investigating whether Anh has been experiencing auditory hallucinations accompanying her seclusive behaviour and her opinion that others speak badly of her.

Anh: Yes.

Tom: Whose voices are they, Anh?

> He goes on to learn more about the details of Anh's belief system and how this belief system may have influenced her perceptions of her social network.

Anh: Tuyet and Hung [Anh's brother-in-law]. They say bad things about me behind my back. They say I am a stupid idiot. They don't want me to be with my husband. They don't want me to be happy. They introduced this girl to my husband and he married her.

> Anh's responses suggest that she may be experiencing auditory hallucinations with paranoid overtones involving her sister's family. She also maintains unrealistic expectations of a reunion with her former fiancé. Anh's developing trust in Tom allows her to disclose information that she is likely to find shameful about her ex-fiancé's abandonment of her.

Tom: Anh, how do you know they introduced someone else to your fiancé?

Anh: I know, I know everything. I have heard everything.

> This response lends weight to the view that Anh's thinking may be delusional.

Tom: I understand you haven't seen Duc [former fiancé] for some years, is that right?

Anh: (nods) He's my fiancé. He will come back to me.

Tom: Why do you think your sister and her husband would be saying these things about you?

> From meetings with Anh's sister Tom has the impression that Tuyet and her husband are generally supportive. However, Tuyet and Hung may be angry with Anh if they believe that Anh is being visited by the spirit of a deceased ancestor that she has offended (the cause). Moreover, they may feel that Anh is bringing the stigma of mental illness on their family. Tom seeks more detail about Anh's relationship with the couple.

Anh: They are bad people; they are very bad.

Tom: Anh, have you had the opportunity to talk to your family in Vietnam, your mother, for example, about this? What do you think she would say if you told her that, when you are alone, you could hear voices speaking to you? What do you think your mother would say about that?

> Here Tom's questions explore two issues. The first is whether the social network may be consulted in dealing with the experience of the "voices" (as part of the question, "What treatments are relevant solutions to the voices?"). The second deals with the cultural interpretation of Anh's

experiences. Are the voices "normal" in her particular circumstances or do others of her cultural background consider her experience extraordinary?

Anh: My mother, I wrote and told her and she didn't believe me. She said that Tuyet is good and she said I have to pray. She said that my grandmother loves me very much and came to talk to me because she missed me when she died.

Tom verifies that those who share Anh's culture do not necessarily share her conviction that hearing voices is normal.

Referring to her mother's view, Anh attempts to reaffirm the similarity between the culturally accepted experience of the voice of the grandmother's ghost and her present experience.

Tom: But your main problem is hearing the voice of Tuyet and Hung, not your grandmother.

However, Tom maintains the distinction. Tom's line of questioning draws on the perspective of the professional model, which is likely to view Anh's experience as a psychotic state. This view is based on accumulating evidence that includes the perspective of Anh's family. He is also subtly preparing Anh to receive a different explanation for her experience by distinguishing it from normal cultural behaviour.

Anh: My mother said my grandmother is very good, she would not say bad things about me. My mother said I have to go to the temple and pray. I went back to the monk and he gave me some amulets.

Anh describes what may be culturally appropriate treatments of prayer and amulets.

Tom: How do the amulets help?

Tom shows respect for this traditional religious treatment and engages Anh's trust further by asking questions that show genuine interest in this practice. His question seeks to understand what the therapeutic/preventative "mechanism of action" is of the amulets.

Anh: I have one to wear around my neck, one to keep in my purse, one to put in the doorway of my room and one on my mirror. They protect me from the bad spirits. They are everywhere and if they see an amulet in front of your house, they go away.

Tom: Have the amulets helped with the voices?

Anh: (softly) No.

Tom: So you are still hearing the voices. Is that right?

> As with the offerings at the temple mentioned earlier, Tom invites Anh to concede that the cultural solution of amulets has not been entirely effective. Or alternatively, has not been effective in ameliorating the voices. This leaves the possibility that it has been effective in other ways. He continues to set the scene for introducing a Western medical model and for negotiating an alternative treatment approach.

Anh: Yes.

Tom: All right. So you are going to the temple here and you are getting amulets, but you are still quite troubled by the ghost and the voices, and you are still quite upset about your fiancé having left you.

> Tom reaffirms that the cultural treatment has had only limited impact on Anh's experiences.

Anh: Yes.

> Through Anh's acknowledgement that she is still troubled despite the traditional treatments, Tom has found common ground, providing a basis for negotiation.

Tom: So do you think as well as going to the temple you need some additional help?

> Instead of saying that the traditional treatment is incapable of helping Anh, Tom proposes a collaborative treatment approach. Here he is attempting to provide a strategy that is *additional* to Anh's.

Anh: Yes.

> The common ground has been extended through Anh's acceptance that she needs additional help.

Tom: As your doctor has discussed with you, he has medication that might help with the voices you are hearing to make them less frequent, or even to make them go away.

Anh: No, no, no.

> Tom will have a tough time convincing Anh of the value of Western medication, given her previous history with it. Although Anh grew up in a high power distance culture, she has responded to Tom's expectation that she will act as an equal in the therapeutic relationship. By objecting to the medication, she is asserting her right to express her views openly, rather than agreeing with him out of respect for his authority as a male and a clinician. Of course, this is also an issue she feels strongly about.

At this point differing explanatory models are held strongly by each participant in the interaction despite Tom's attempts to draw Anh's attention to the limited effectiveness of her model.

Tom: So what is your objection to that?

Tom now attempts to examine the basis for Anh's response.

Anh: My mum said the medication is poison.

Tom discovers that the family has their own formulation of the nature of Western medicines previously tried and he needs to understand what this formulation is. Tom is reminded here that, in the context of a collectivist culture, he is negotiating the Western model with Anh *and* her family.

Tom: So, what has been explained to you about the medication Anh? What do you know about it?

Rather than insisting on the value and efficacy of psychotropic medication, Tom investigates what her objections might be. Some of the symptoms Anh describes below may be side-effects of excessive medication.[3]

Anh: It gives me a backache, a stomachache, a headache and it's causing me to shake like this and I have to walk up and down, up and down.

Anh's responses reveal that a series of uncomfortable physical experiences, in addition to family reactions (to deal with the medication), form the basis of Anh's objections.

Tom: You believe that is connected to taking the medication do you?

Tom does not assume that Anh is "just somatising" but takes her complaints seriously.

Anh: Yes. The medication is too hot, my mum said, no medication, my mum said. She threw it out when I visited her in Vietnam.

Anh's reference to the hot qualities of medication is related to the Taoist belief that hot and cold elements in the body should be in balance. Tom investigates this a little later.

Tom: Anh, the reason why we are suggesting medication is because we think the voices are caused by an illness. From what you have said, you are obviously very upset about losing your fiancé and your grandmother, and your reactions to those things seem to be quite normal. Many people are visited by ghosts, in

---

3 People of Asian background tend to require lower doses of psychotropic medication (Lambert & Minas, 1998).

your culture, when someone dies, but these voices are different. We believe that these voices are related to an illness that you have, that we can treat.

> This is Tom's attempt at conveying the Western explanatory model of mental illness in lay language. He reaffirms to Anh the value of medication and that the professional model regards medication to be useful in ameliorating voices. At the same time Tom acknowledges Anh's losses and her attempt to give meaning to her distressing experiences by attributing them to culturally accepted sources.

Anh: Ghosts are everywhere; everybody believes that there are ghosts everywhere.

> At this point it seems that Anh is unconvinced by Tom's explanatory model and maintains her own model, which "makes better sense" of the distressing experiences she is suffering.

Tom: These voices don't seem to be going away even though you have been going to the temple. The medication is used to try and get rid of those voices. Now you've said that you don't want to take …

> However, Tom wishes to establish whether (if the side-effects could be controlled) there have been any benefits from the medication that Anh might acknowledge.

Anh: No, no. It makes my skin swollen. I am shaking and I have to walk up and down and my sister says that I look stupid, walking up and down, up and down. No. No medication. It's poisonous.

Tom: All right, you've told me three objections to the medication. One is that it makes you physically uncomfortable, secondly, your mother doesn't agree with it, and thirdly, you said it was too hot. What do you mean by that?

> Tom reaches a momentary stalemate with Anh, but he moves to address the issues of physical discomfort that he originally passed over. He does not contest the view of Anh and her mother that medication is poisonous, but instead acknowledges the distress it causes Anh. In summarising her objections to the medication Tom accepts that there is validity to her objections (rather than dismissing them as mere "non-compliance"). Tom adopts the term "too hot" used by Anh to describe her experiences in a way that is culturally meaningful to her. This reaffirms the collaborative relationship as Tom explores what implications the Western medication has within Anh's explanatory model. During this process Tom learns about the cultural concept of hot and the means of managing hot states.

Anh: It is too hot. When I went to Vietnam my mum made me eat a lot of tofu and vegetables because the medication is too hot. It makes me feel too hot.

> Tom knows something about the hot and cold qualities of food and medicines and that they are associated with the yin and yang elements that need to be in balance for the harmonious functioning of the universe and the body. But, by asking Anh to explain these ideas to him, he is demonstrating that his understanding and hers may not be the same. He is also showing that *his* knowledge of the cultural belief is not what is important, but the interpretation and meaning that Anh places on that belief in the context of her complaints. This may provide him with a means to make the medication more acceptable to Anh.

Tom: So when a medication is too hot, it makes you feel too hot. What other effects does it have? When something is too hot, how does that affect you?

> Tom finds out whether there are similar substances that have similar effects to psychotropic medicines and what is done to counter these effects. This information may also be useful in countering the hot effects of medication.

Anh: I can't go to the toilet, I get pimples all over my face. It is very bad. It's very hot so that I can't sleep, you know.

Tom: Anh, are there other things that are too hot and have this effect on the body?

Anh: Chocolate, coffee.

Tom: Is there anything you can do about — if something is too hot, or your body is affected in this way — is there anything you can do about it? Do you have any treatment for that?

Anh: My mum cooks green beans and you have to drink a lot of water. You should not have a lot of chocolate. So if you don't take medication you are OK.

Tom: Anh, if we could find a medication that wasn't going to give you these side-effects, and if you treated yourself for the heat that is caused by the medication by eating these things, would you consider trying it for a little while to see if it reduced the voices?

> Tom uses what he has learnt from Anh to reintroduce a collaborative treatment strategy using both Western and traditional treatments. This model offers Anh a solution to the voices and invites her to use her own cultural strategies to manage the apparent side-effects of medication.

Anh: I did. I tried the medication before. It didn't work. I took it, and it didn't work.

Tom: When you say it didn't work did it have any effect on the voices at all or not? Did it reduce the voices at all?

Anh: Um, yes.

> By obtaining Anh's agreement that, despite the unpleasant side-effects, the medication did reduce the voices, Tom has the means to negotiate treatment. He suggests that side-effects can be reduced while traditional treatment can be used to reduce the "hotness" of medication, thereby accommodating Western treatment to the client's framework.

Tom: So it did reduce them? Would you agree that it would be good to get rid of these voices?

Anh: They're too noisy. I can't sleep; they talk about me all the time.

Tom: Yes. But you don't want to be having all these side-effects. There may be something we can do about this. If it's all right with you, I'll talk to your doctor about this. If the medication controls the voices, you might be able to sleep better too. What I would like is for you to continue to visit the temple so that you can also get your own kind of treatment.

> By endorsing Anh's visits to the temple Tom is showing genuine respect for this traditional treatment approach, is giving it clinical validation and is acknowledging what is important for her.

Anh: OK. If it will help me sleep … Can you help me to get my fiancé back? It's my fate, you know. I am meant to be his wife.

> Tom and Anh have reached an agreement that something can be done and have created for Anh a sense of having some choices and some control over what happens to her. Once the more immediate issue of medication is resolved, the underlying issue of Anh's preoccupation with her former fiancé re-emerges. Tom has achieved credibility by showing respect for her explanatory model and by providing benefit (i.e., assuring her that the voices can be controlled without unpleasant side-effects). Having achieved credibility, Anh now wants to know if Tom can return her fiancé to her.

Tom: That's something we need to talk more about, trying to sort out what went wrong there. Do you think that the monk can help you with matters of your fate?

> Tom responds both in terms of his own framework (interpersonal problems can be solved by talking about them) and Anh's explanatory model, which implicates fate. What solutions do her explanatory model offer?

Anh: I need to go back to the temple in Vietnam to change my fate.

The process of negotiation illustrated in this transcript is an ongoing process throughout the duration of the clinical relationship. Occasions for negotiation may occur during assessment, during psychotherapy and during discharge planning. Although Tom found common ground and reached a shared agreement regarding treatment with Anh, it should not be assumed that Anh's conceptualisation of her condition will remain static. Tom may need to reframe the shared understanding as Anh's explanatory model undergoes changes as a result of her therapeutic relationship with Tom, through her contact with psychiatric rehabilitation services and through her increased contact with the English-speaking community. As explained earlier in this chapter, an individual's explanatory model may undergo rapid change once contact with the medical system occurs and during the process of acculturation (Angel & Thoits, 1987).

Anh: A Culturally Sensitive Clinical Formulation

We have discussed many issues that relate to the assessment of the mental health of a person from a culture different to that of the clinicians. We will now illustrate how these issues may enter a clinical formulation.

A standard clinical formulation represents a conceptualisation of the case that provides an account of factors contributing to the disorder and proposes hypothetical connections between the client's experiences and their illness (Dakis & Singh, 1994). A cultural formulation should similarly aspire to describe "etiological determinants, including predisposing, precipitating and perpetuating factors and biopsychosocial influences ... brought together to make sense of the case beyond the level of summary and diagnosis" (Dakis & Singh, 1994, p. 93). What is not made explicit in this definition, however, is that relevant cultural factors should be integrated into each part of a formulation. For this reason the term "culturally sensitive clinical formulation" may be preferred because it implies that cultural information is integral to the clinical formulation, rather than being added on as a separate attachment. It also acts to remind clinicians that cultural factors need to be considered in every aspect of a mental health assessment. As suggested in DSM-IV, and as described in detail at the end of chapter 1, a culturally sensitive clinical formulation should make reference to the issues enumerated below. Although these factors do not need to be addressed in the following sequence, the formulation should make reference to:

- the client's cultural identity

- cultural explanations of the illness

- cultural factors related to psychosocial environment and levels of functioning

- migration history (for refugees, migrants or for people whose parents were refugees or migrants)

- cultural elements of the relationship between the person and the clinician
- overall cultural assessment and formulation for diagnosis and care.

In the culturally sensitive formulation of Anh's case that follows, the cultural features of her case are explained explicitly. Clinicians may not always wish to include this degree of detail in every aspect of the formulation, but it should be kept in mind that the formulation is a communication to other clinicians who may not understand the implications of the cultural issues you may describe.

Anh's Formulation

Anh is a single 30-year-old Vietnamese woman who speaks English at a low-to-moderate level of proficiency. This level of English proficiency indicates that she would be unable to discuss clinical issues in English and, therefore, she was interviewed with a qualified interpreter to ensure accurate two-way communication. The interpreter was known to Anh which, in this case, enhanced trust. Anh migrated to Australia in 1994 to marry a Vietnamese man who had sponsored her. He rejected her when she was diagnosed with paranoid schizophrenia in 1995. Anh has been treated with haloperidol for auditory hallucinations and paranoid delusions at her local mental health service but moved into our catchment area recently. She was on a compulsory community treatment order because she refused to take her medication. Anh has been living with her married sister, her brother-in-law and their two children and these family members are an important source of support for Anh.

Anh's childhood was unsettled as she grew up during the Vietnam War, but she has said little of any trauma she and her family may have suffered during the war. Nevertheless, it is important to be alert for possible signs of posttraumatic stress disorder or other symptoms related to her war and post-war experiences. Following the war Anh suffered the loss of her father (who was in the South Vietnamese army), when he died in a re-education camp. As Anh was sponsored to migrate to Australia by her former fiancé she did not undergo the hardships that refugees from Vietnam experienced; however, she has had to face the stresses of resettlement and adaptation to a culture very different to her own. These stresses include the language barrier, differing cultural values and beliefs, and separation from important members of her family. Significant people left behind when she migrated included her mother and three siblings, as well as a large extended family. Her mother is particularly significant to her. They write regularly to each other, and her mother is influential in Anh's cooperation with treatment.

Anh's sister works as a child support worker and the family is reasonably supportive of Anh. However, there are culturally-based role expectations that Anh, as a younger sister, help with housework. Stresses initially occurred when Anh was unwell and unable to help, thereby failing to meet cultural norms of daily functioning.

Anh also places pressure on herself to meet cultural role expectations. However, the sister has developed an understanding of Anh's illness through her contact with mental health services, has lowered her expectations, and appreciates the support provided by the service. Anh's sister is not aware of any history of mental illness in the family. It cannot be assumed that the sister conceptualises Anh's problem as a mental illness. The visits to the temple by both Anh and her sister suggest that the sister may regard Anh's problem within the limits of normality, or may be attempting to normalise Anh's problem as one of spirit possession, resembling their experiences following the grandmother's death.

Anh has not been employed since she became ill and tends to be socially withdrawn, with no friends beyond those of her sister's circle. Anh's predominant cultural identity is likely to be Vietnamese, as she was born in Vietnam and her reference groups are Vietnamese people in Australia (that is, her sister's family) and her family in Vietnam. In addition, she prefers to speak Vietnamese and nominates her ethnic identity as Vietnamese. She has acculturated to Australian society to only a limited extent because she has not formed close relationships with Australians through work or social activities. A source of psychosocial stress may be Anh's cultural identity as an unmarried Vietnamese woman aged in her 30s. This role tends to be stigmatised in Vietnamese society, possibly contributing to Anh's social isolation. Her continuing preoccupation with her former fiancé could also be understood in this context.

There may be further stigma associated with Anh's identity as a person with a mental illness. The extreme stigma associated with mental illness in Vietnamese society may help to explain why Anh was rejected by her fiancé. Anh therefore carries the double stigma of being an older single woman and having a mental illness. These conceptions of herself may be associated with her diminished self-esteem and confidence. In addition, both are likely to have contributed to her being lonely and alienated from her community. Anh (and her sister) also lacks the social supports of her extended family, upon which great reliance would be placed in Vietnam. Instead, heavy demands are placed on her sister's family. Because Anh has a mental illness, the community may blame her and her family. Her sister's family may therefore see her as a burden and someone to be hidden from the community. In reality, the family appears to be supportive, but it cannot be assumed that there is no ambivalence.

The burden on Anh and on her sister is to some extent relieved by the spiritual support provided to both by their strong belief in Buddhism and together they visit a Buddhist temple regularly.

In her initial relationship with the male clinician Anh avoided eye contact and showed a reluctance to speak. This may have been due to anxiety. However, it could also have been a sign of deference given that in Vietnam it is not considered polite to speak first or to speak up when in the presence of someone who is considered to be of higher status. Initially Anh insisted on calling the psychologist "doctor", as she was unfamiliar with the role of psychologist. The interpersonal dynamics of the clinical relationship have been negotiated so that more recently Anh has accepted the invitation to call the clinician by his first name. She has also allowed him to use her first name after he asked how she wished to be addressed. As the therapeutic relationship has developed over the last of couple of months Anh's confidence and trust has increased and she has been more willing to discuss her beliefs and personal feelings.

The auditory hallucinations for which Anh has been treated can be distinguished into two kinds. In the past she has heard the voice of her deceased grandmother speaking to her, which appears to be a culturally accepted idiom of distress when a loved family member has died. Anh's sister has also heard this voice and they have sought the help of the temple (a culturally approved treatment) to settle the ghost. As the grandmother died 2 years ago Anh acknowledges that the voices she has been hearing more recently have been the voices of a different ghost and of her sister and her brother-in-law saying negative things about her. When Anh wrote to her mother about these voices her mother expressed her disapproval of Anh's beliefs and directed her to seek help at the temple.

Anh has not taken the treatment prescribed by the previous mental health service as she complains that it caused multiple physical symptoms, which are consistent with the range of side-effects expected from the medication. The treatment was also not consistent with the explanatory model of the family (particularly her mother), which added to Anh's reluctance to adhere to it. When Anh visited Vietnam, her mother expressed disapproval of the medication, saying it was too "hot" from the perspective of Chinese medicine and labelling it "poison". Nevertheless, Anh acknowledged that medication had reduced the incidence of the voices.

As people of Asian background tend to require lower doses of psychotropic medication the treatment plan is to review whether the level of medication is appropriate for Anh to ensure that side-effects are minimised. Anh's community treatment order is to be lifted as she has agreed to take medication while continuing with traditional treatments, including visits to the Buddhist temple for amulets and prayers. To address the "hot" quality of medication, and to restore the balance of yin and yang in the body, Anh advises that she needs to eat green vegetables and drink a lot of water. She reports that she is not taking any herbal medications, therefore there should be no risks of interaction with neuroleptic medication. In collectivist cultures, the support and cooperation of the family is vital in successfully implementing treatment. For this reason the treatment plan will be discussed with the sister and, with her and Anh's agreement, a letter will be written to the mother explaining the treatment and its rationale. This letter acknowledges the important role Anh's mother plays in her life and treatment, and also addresses the mother's concerns. The negotiated treatment plan incorporates both Western and traditional treatment, addressing the explanatory models of the client, the client's family (in Australia and Vietnam) and the clinician.

In future sessions, Anh's preoccupation with her former fiancé will be discussed to determine whether she can come to terms with this loss. She will be seen weekly for psychotherapy and for monitoring of her mental state. To further develop the therapeutic relationship the meaning and personal implications for Anh of the "hot" and "cold" elements in Chinese medicine will continue to be explored. Anh plans to visit a temple in Vietnam to try to change the fate that she is destined to marry this man. Belief in the influence of fate is culturally normative. This trip will also provide her with an opportunity to visit her mother.

Postscript: Clinical Outcome for Anh

As described in chapter 6, Anh visited Vietnam some months later and followed the ritual at the Buddhist temple to change her fate. The message in the temple wall predicted a different fate than that she was to marry her fiancé, and when she returned to Australia she had lost her preoccupation with Duc.

Adjusted dosage of medication controlled Anh's auditory hallucinations, as well as the side-effects she was experiencing. She has become less isolative and has been attending a psychiatric rehabilitation program. She has expressed interest in visiting an employment support service, with a view to eventually gaining a part-time job.

An important function of a comprehensive culturally sensitive cultural formulation is to communicate to other clinicians the cultural factors important in understanding the client. This is to ensure that these factors are not overlooked if the treating clinician leaves, or if the client comes into contact with other facets of the mental health service, such as the crisis team or the inpatient unit.

Conclusion

In this chapter we have endeavoured to draw together a number of the issues raised in the various chapters of this book as they may be seen in an individual case. In particular, Anh's case illustrated how cultural beliefs regarding spirit possession influenced her conceptualisation of her illness. The interview demonstrated how her explanatory model was gradually elicited, how culturally normative beliefs were distinguished from symptoms of mental illness and how the clinician's explanatory model was explained to, but not imposed on the client. Anh's and her family's explanatory models did not match that of the clinician. However, the interview provided an example of the way in which discrepancies between explanatory models can be negotiated so that treatment is implemented to manage distressing experiences and behaviours. At the same time, the clinician acknowledged and showed respect for the client's worldview during the interview and accommodated traditional treatment that is consistent with that world-view. Anh's case also showed the central role that the family may play in collectivist cultures in implementing and maintaining treatment. Finally, the information elicited from Anh was integrated into a culturally sensitive clinical formulation that contained enough information on cultural issues relevant to Anh's mental health to inform other clinicians.

Conclusion

In the course of this book people from a number of different cultures have been encountered, each with different problems. What they had in common was that their problems and symptoms did not fit the diagnostic categories of the DSM-IV. Their symptoms tended to be of a kind rarely reported by people of a Western background. Samuel, of Nigerian background, complained of crawling sensations in his head and of having been bewitched; Lin, born in China, believed she was a ghost and a bad person, and would not return to China because her academic failure would "kill her family"; Thuy, from Vietnam, described a range of affective and somatic symptoms that spanned diagnostic boundaries; Danny and his family, who were of Lebanese background, attributed his deterioration in functioning to the evil eye; Hong, who came from Vietnam was suicidal and believed she and her son were possessed by spirits; while Anh, also born in Vietnam, reported that she was hearing the voice of her beloved dead grandmother. The stories of each of these people have shown that applying a Western diagnostic framework would distort their illness experience. Briefer case vignettes also illustrated the potential for misdiagnosis for people from a number of other cultures.

We have demonstrated that misdiagnosis and inappropriate treatment can only be avoided through an exploration of the cultural and psychosocial background of each client. Specifically, this involves a thoughtful evaluation of the clinician's values and the client's cultural values; an awareness of cultural differences in expression and communication of affect; and a respectful and empathic investigation of the client's and family's explanatory model of their problem. It is this comprehensive crosscultural investigation and self-scrutiny that comprises the individual cultural approach that we first discussed in chapter 1.

In this book we have endeavoured to provide the clinician with a framework for obtaining an in-depth understanding of a client whose cultural background is different from their own. We have not attempted to resolve major theoretical debates; for example, what the relative contributions of biology and culture are to the different manifestations of mental illness across cultures. Rather, to help clinicians avoid misdiagnosis and plan appropriate treatment we have highlighted the crosscultural differences that do exist. And rather than providing a comprehensive account of every cultural belief system a clinician may encounter, we have described two major belief systems and illustrated how such belief systems can impact on an individual's views of health and illness. We also have provided strategies to elicit the beliefs and explanatory models of clients from other cultures.

In essence, we have tried to demonstrate that the methods of Western mental health practice are tied to a Western cultural world-view and to Western manifestations of mental illness. Not surprisingly then, non-Western expressions of mental illness may not fit the Western model. We hope that this book will encourage clinicians to suspend preconceived diagnostic classifications to conduct an emic study of the client's illness experience.

References

Adebimpe, V.R. (1981). Overview: White norms and psychiatric diagnosis of black patients. *American Journal of Psychiatry, 138,* 279–285.

Akighir, A. (1982). Traditional and modern psychiatry: A survey of opinions and beliefs amongst people in Plateau State, Nigeria. *International Journal of Social Psychiatry, 28,* 203–209.

Alarcon, R.D. (1995). Culture and psychiatric diagnosis: Impact on DSM-IV and ICD-10. *The Psychiatric Clinics of North America, 18,* 449–465.

Al Krenawi, A. (1999). Explanations of mental health symptoms by the Bedouin-Arabs of the Negev. *International Journal of Social Psychiatry, 45,* 56–64.

American Psychiatric Association. (1987). *Diagnostic and statistical manual of mental disorders* (3rd ed. rev.). Washington: Author.

American Psychiatric Association. (1994). *Diagnostic and statistical manual of mental disorders* (4th ed.). Washington: Author.

Angel, R., & Thoits, P. (1987). The impact of culture on the cognitive structure of illness. *Culture, Medicine and Psychiatry, 11,* 465–494.

Bagulho, F., & Chiu, E. (1997). Translations of Folstein's Mini-Mental State Examination. *Connections: Newsletter of the Victorian Transcultural Mental Health Network. February,* 1–2.

Baker, R., & Briggs, J. (1975). Working with interpreters in social work practice. *Australian Social Work, 28,* 31–37.

Barrett, R.J. (1997). Cultural formulation of psychiatric diagnosis. Death on a horse's back: Adjustment disorder with panic attacks. *Culture, Medicine and Psychiatry, 21,* 481–496.

Becker, G. (1994). Swallowing frogs: Anger and illness in Northeast Brazil. *Medical Anthropology Quarterly, 8,* 360–382.

Bhatia, M.S., & Malik, S.C. (1991). Dhat syndrome — A useful diagnostic entity in Indian culture. *British Journal of Psychiatry, 159,* 691–695.

Bhurga, D., & Bhui, K. (1997). Clinical management of patients across cultures. *Advances in Psychiatric Treatment, 3,* 233–239.

Bontempo, R. (1993). Translation fidelity of psychological scales: An item response theory analysis of an individualism–collectivism scale. *Journal of Cross-Cultural Psychology, 24,* 149–166.

Brav, A. (1981). The evil eye among the Hebrews. In A. Dundes (Ed.), *The evil eye: A folklore casebook* (pp. 44–54). New York: Garland.

Brown L. (Ed.). (1993). *The new shorter Oxford English dictionary on historical principles.* Oxford: Clarendon Press.

Campbell, R.J. (1996). *Psychiatric dictionary* (7th ed.). Oxford: Oxford University Press.

Casson, R. (1983). Schemata in cognitive anthropology. *Annual Review of Anthropology, 12,* 429–462.

Cheung, F.M. (1995). Facts and myths about somatisation among the Chinese. In T-Y. Lin, W-S. Tseng & E-K. Yeh (Eds.), *Chinese societies and mental health* (pp. 156–166). Hong Kong: Oxford University Press.

Cheung, F., & Lin, K.M. (1997). Neurasthenia, depression and somatoform disorder in a Chinese-Vietnamese woman migrant. *Culture, Medicine and Psychiatry, 21,* 247–258.

Chinese Culture Connection. (1987). Chinese values and the search for a culture free dimension of culture. *Journal of Cross-Cultural Psychology, 18,* 143–164.

Chinnery, J. (1996a). Confucianism. In C. Scott Littleton (Ed.), *The sacred East: Hinduism, Buddhism, Confucianism, Daoism, Shinto* (pp. 92–115). Melbourne, Australia: Cardigan Street Publishers.

Chinnery, J. (1996b). Daoism. In C. Scott Littleton (Ed.), *The sacred East: Hinduism, Buddhism, Confucianism, Daoism, Shinto* (pp. 116–143). Melbourne Australia: Cardigan Street Publishers.

Choca, J.P., Shanley, L.A., Peterson, C.A., & Van Denburg, E. (1990). Racial bias and the MCMI. *Journal of Personality Assessment, 54,* 479–490.

Chung-yuan, C. (1963). *Creativity and taoism: A study of Chinese philosophy, art and poetry.* New York: Harper & Row.

Collins, J., Stolk, Y., Saunders, T., Garlick, R., Stankovska, M., & Lynagh, M. (2002). *I feel so sad it breaks my heart: The Mid West NESB carers' project.* Melbourne: NorthWestern Mental Health.

Corin, E. (1996). Cultural comments on organic and psychotic disorders: I. In J.E. Mezzich, A. Kleinman, H. Fabrega & D.L. Parron (Eds.), *Culture and Psychiatric Diagnosis: A DSM-IV Perspective* (pp. 63–69). Washington: American Psychiatric Press.

Dakis, J., & Singh, B.S. (1994). Making sense of the psychiatric patient. In S. Bloch & B.S. Singh (Eds.), *Foundations of clinical psychiatry* (pp. 79–96). Melbourne: Melbourne University Press.

D'Andrade, R. (1990). Some propositions about the relations between culture and human cognition. In J.W. Stigler, R.A. Shweder & G. Herdt (Eds.), *Cultural psychology: Essays on comparative human development* (pp. 65–129). Cambridge: Cambridge University Press.

Dein, S., & Lipsedge, M. (1998). Negotiating across class, culture and religion: Psychiatry in the English inner city. In S.O. Okpaku (Ed.), *Clinical methods in transcultural psychiatry* (pp. 137–154). Washington: American Psychiatric Press.

Del Castillo, J.C. (1970). The influence of language upon symtomatology in foreign-born patients. *American Journal of Psychiatry, 127,* 242–244.

Dinh, T. (1998). *Working with the Vietnamese community.* Melbourne: South West Area Mental Health Service.

Donaldson, B.A. (1981). The evil eye in Iran. In A. Dundes (Ed.), *The evil eye: A folklore casebook* (pp. 66–77). New York: Garland.

Draguns, J.G. (1989a). Dilemmas and choices in cross-cultural counselling: The universal versus the culturally distinctive. In P.B. Pedersen, J.G. Draguns, W.J. Lonner & J.E. Trimble (Eds.), *Counselling across cultures.* (pp. 3–21). Honolulu: University of Hawaii Press.

Draguns, J.G. (1989b). Normal and abnormal behaviour in cross-cultural perspective: Specifying the nature of their relationship. In J. Berman (Ed.), *Nebraska symposium on motivation* (pp. 235–277). Lincoln: University of Nebraska Press.

Dundes, A. (1981). Wet and dry, the evil eye: An essay in Indo-European and Semitic worldview. In A. Dundes (Ed.), *The evil eye: A folklore casebook* (pp. 257–298). New York: Garland.

Durkheim, E. (1970). *Suicide: A study in sociology.* (J.A. Spaulding & G. Simpson, Trans.). London: Routledge & Kegan Paul. (Original work published 1897.)

Ebden, P., Bhatt, A., Carey, O.J. & Harrison, B. (1988). The bilingual consultation. *The Lancet, February,* 347.

Ebigbo, P.O. (1982). Development of a culture specific (Nigeria) screening scale of somatic complaints indicating psychiatric disturbance. *Culture, Medicine and Psychiatry, 6,* 29–43.

Eisenbruch, M. (1990). Classification of natural and supernatural causes of mental distress: Development of a mental distress explanatory model questionnaire. *Journal of Nervous and Mental Disease, 178,* 712–719.

Elworthy, F.T. (1989). *The evil eye: An account of this ancient and widespread superstition.* New York: Bell Publishing Company.

Escobar, J.I. (1987) Cross-cultural aspects of the somatization trait. *Hospital and Community Psychiatry, 38,* 174–180.

Fabrega, H. (1987). Psychiatric diagnosis: A cultural perspective. *The Journal of Nervous and Mental Disease, 175,* 383–393.

Fabrega, H. (1989). The self and schizophrenia: A cultural perspective. *Schizophrenia Bulletin, 15,* 277–290.

Fabrega, H. (1991). Psychiatric stigma in non-Western societies. *Comprehensive Psychiatry, 32,* 534–551.

Fadiman, A. (1997). *The spirit catches you and you fall down.* New York: Farrar, Strauss & Giroux.

Farmer, A.E., & Falkowski, W. (1985). Maggot in the salt, the snake factor and the treatment of atypical psychosis in West-African women. *British Journal of Psychiatry, 146,* 446–448.

Fitzpatrick, R. (1984). Lay concepts of illness. In R. Fitzpatrick, J. Hinton, S. Newman, G. Scambler & J. Thompson (Eds.), *The experience of illness* (pp. 11–31). London: Tavistock.

Flaherty, J.A., Gavira, M., Pathak, D., Mitchell, T., Wintrob, R., Richman, J.A., et al. (1988). Developing instruments for cross-cultural psychiatric research. *Journal of Nervous and Mental Disease, 176*, 257–263.

Fortescue, M. (1984). *West Greenlandic.* London: Dover

Gaines, A.D. (1982). Cultural definitions, behavior and the person in American psychiatry. In A.J. Marsella & G.M. White (Eds.), *Cultural conceptions of mental health and therapy* (pp. 167–192). Dordrecht: Reidel.

Gauld, A., & Shotter, J. (1977). *Human action and its psychological investigation.* London: Routledge & Kegan Paul.

Giddens, A. (1972) *Emile Durkheim: Selected writings.* London: Cambridge University Press.

Gil, J. (1998). *Metamorpheses of the body.* Minneapolis: University of Minnesota Press.

Gillis, L.S., Elk, R., Ben, A., & Teggin, A. (1982). The present state examination: Experiences with Xhosa-speaking psychiatric patients. *British Journal of Psychiatry, 141*, 43–147.

Good, B.J. (1993). Culture, diagnosis and comorbidity. *Culture, Medicine and Psychiatry, 16*, 1–20.

Good, B.J. (1996a). Culture and DSM-IV: Diagnosis, knowledge and power. *Culture, Medicine and Psychiatry, 20*, 127–132.

Good, B.J. (1996b). Epilogue: knowledge, power and diagnosis. In J.E. Mezzich, A. Kleinman, H. Fabrega & D.L. Parron (Eds.), *Culture and psychiatric diagnosis: A DSM-IV perspective* (pp. 347–351). Washington: American Psychiatric Press.

Good, B.J., & Good, M.D. (1982). Toward a meaning-centred analysis of popular illness categories: "Fright illness" and "heart distress" in Iran. In A.J. Marsella & G.M. White (Eds.), *Cultural conceptions of mental health and therapy* (pp. 141–166). Dordrecht: Reidel.

Good, B.J., Good, M.D., & Moradi, R. (1985). The interpretation of Iranian depressive illness and dysphoric affect. In A. Kleinman, B.J. Good (Eds.), *Culture and depression: Studies in the anthropology and cross-cultural psychiatry of affect and disorder* (pp. 369–428). Berkeley: University of California Press.

Gotlib, I.H., & McCabe, S.B. (1992). An information-processing approach to the study of cognitive functioning in depression. In E.F. Walker, R.H. Dworkin & B.A. Cornblatt (Eds.), *Experimental personality and psychopathology research* (pp. 131–161). New York: Springer.

Graham, E.A., & Chitnarong, J. (1997). Ethnographic study among Seattle Cambodians: Wind illness. *Ethnomed.* Retrieved 20 November, 1998, from http://www.healthlinks.washington.edu/clinical/ethnomed/ethno_wind.html

Griffith, E.H. (1996). African American perspectives. In J.E. Mezzich, A. Kleinman, H. Fabrega & D.L. Parron (Eds.), *Culture and psychiatric diagnosis: A DSM-IV perspective* (pp. 27–29). Washington: American Psychiatric Press.

Guarnaccia, P.J., Rubio-Stipec, M., & Canino, G.J. (1989). Ataques de nervios in the Puerto Rico Diagnostic Interview Schedule: The impact of cultural categories on psychiatric epidemiology. *Culture, Medicine and Psychiatry, 13,* 275–295.

Guinness, E.A. (1992a). III. Profile and prevalence of the brain fag syndrome: Psychiatric morbidity in school populations in Africa. *British Journal of Psychiatry, 160,* 42–52.

Guinness, E.A. (1992b). IV. Social origins of the brain fag syndrome. *British Journal of Psychiatry, 160,* 53–64.

Hardie, M.M. (1981) The evil eye in some Greek villages. In A. Dundes (Ed.), *The evil eye: A folklore casebook* (pp. 107–123). New York: Garland.

Harfouche, J.K. (1981) The evil eye and infant health in Lebanon. In A. Dundes (Ed.), *The evil eye: A folklore casebook* (pp. 86–106). New York: Garland.

Harris, B. (1981). A case of brain fag in East Africa. *British Journal of Psychiatry, 138,* 162–163.

Health and Community Services. (1994). *Victoria's mental health services: Improved access through co-ordinated client care.* Melbourne: Psychiatric Services Branch.

Health and Community Services. (1995). *Victoria's mental health services consumer information guide: How case management can help you.* Melbourne: Psychiatric Services Division.

Helman, C.G. (1984). *Culture, health and illness.* London: John Wright & Sons.

Herzfeld, M. (1986). Closure as cure: Tropes in the exploration of bodily and social disorder. *Current Anthropology, 27,* 107–120.

Hofstede, G. (1980). *Culture's consequences: International differences in work-related values.* London: Sage Publications.

Hofstede, G. (1991). *Cultures and organizations: Software of the mind.* London: Harper Collins.

Hughes, C.C. (1996). The culture-bound syndromes and psychiatric diagnosis. In J.E. Mezzich, A. Kleinman, H. Fabrega & D.L. Parron (Eds.), *Culture and psychiatric diagnosis: A DSM-IV perspective* (pp. 289–307). Washington: American Psychiatric Press.

Human Services. (1996). *Victoria's mental health services: Improving services for people from a non-English-speaking background.* Melbourne: Psychiatric Services Branch, Victorian Government Department of Human Services.

Ingram, R.E., & Kendall, P.C. (1986). Cognitive clinical psychology: implications of an information processing perspective. In R.E. Ingram (Ed.), *Information processing approaches in clinical psychology* (pp. 4–21). Orlando: Academic Press.

Jablensky, A., Sartorius, N., Ernberg, G., Anker, M., Korten, A., Cooper, J.E., et al. (1992). Schizophrenia: Manifestations, incidence, and course in different cultures. *Psychological Medicine Monograph Supplement 20.*

Jablensky, A., Sartorius, N., Gulbinat, W., & Ernberg, G. (1981). Characteristics of depressive patients contacting psychiatric services in four cultures: A report from the WHO collaborative study on the assessment of depressive disorders. *Acta Psychiatrica Scandinavia, 63,* 367–383.

Jenkins, J.H, Kleinman, A., & Good, B.J. (1991). Cross-cultural studies of depression. In J. Becker & A. Kleinman (Eds.), *Psychosocial aspects of depression* (pp. 67–99). Hillsdale, New Jersey: Lawrence Erlbaum.

Jones, B.E., & Gray, B.A. (1986). Problems in diagnosing schizophrenia and affective disorders among blacks. *Hospital and Community Psychiatry, 37,* 61–65.

Juola, J.F. (1986). Cognitive psychology and information processing: Content and process analysis for a psychology of mind. In R.E. Ingram (Ed.), *Information processing approaches in clinical psychology* (pp. 51–74). Orlando: Academic Press.

Kaplan, H.I., Sadock, B.J., & Grebb, J.A. (1994) *Kaplan and Sadock's synopsis of psychiatry* (7th ed.). Baltimore: William & Wilkins.

Khai, B. (1994). How to say "you" in Vietnamese. In X.T. Nguyen (Ed.), *Vietnamese studies in a multicultural world* (pp. 81–86). Melbourne: Vietnamese Language and Culture Publications.

Kinzie, L.J., & Manson, S.M. (1987). The use of self-rating scales in cross-cultural psychiatry. *Hospital and Community Psychiatry, 38,* 190–196.

Kirmayer, L.J. (1992). The body's insistence on meaning: Metaphor as presentation and representation in illness experience. *Medical Anthropology Quarterly, 6,* 323–346.

Kirmayer, L.J. (1996). Cultural comments on somatoform and dissociative disorders. In J.E. Mezzich, A. Kleinman, H. Fabrega, & D.L. Parron (Eds.), *Culture and psychiatric diagnosis: A DSM-IV perspective* (pp. 151–159). Washington DC: American Psychiatric Press Inc.

Kirmayer, L.J., & Robbins, J.M. (1991). Functional somatic syndromes. In L.J. Kirmayer & J.M. Robbins (Eds.), *Current concepts of somatization: Research and clinical perspectives* (pp. 79–106). Washington DC: American Psychiatric Press.

Kirmayer, L.J., Young, A., & Hayton, B.C. (1995). The cultural context of anxiety disorders. *The Psychiatric Clinics of North America, 18,* 503–521.

Kirmayer, L.J., Young, A., & Robbins, J.M. (1994). Symptom attribution in cultural perspective. *Canadian Journal of Psychiatry, 39,* 584–595.

Kleinman, A. (1980). *Patients and healers in the context of culture: An exploration of the borderland between anthropology, medicine and psychiatry.* Berkeley: University of California Press.

Kleinman, A. (1982). The teaching of clinically applied medical anthropology on a psychiatric consultation-liaison service. In N.J. Chrisman & T.W. Maretzki (Eds.), *Clinically applied anthropology* (pp. 83–115). Dordrecht: Reidel.

Kleinman, A. (1986). *Social origins of distress and disease: Depression, neurasthenia and pain in modern China.* New Haven, CT: Yale University Press.

Kleinman, A. (1988). *Rethinking psychiatry: From cultural category to personal experience.* New York: Free Press.

Kleinman, A. (1996). How is culture important for DSM-IV? In J.E. Mezzich, A. Kleinman, H. Fabrega & D.L. Parron (Eds.), *Culture and psychiatric diagnosis: A DSM-IV perspective* (pp. 15–25). Washington: American Psychiatric Press.

Kleinman, A., Eisenberg, L., & Good, B. (1978). Culture, illness and care: clinical lessons from anthropologic and cross-cultural research. *Annals of Internal Medicine, 88,* 251–258.

Kleinman, A., & Kleinman, J. (1991). Suffering and its professional transformation: Towards and ethnography of interpersonal experience. *Culture Medicine and Psychiatry, 15,* 275–301.

Klimidis, S., Baycan, S., & Punch, J. (2000). *Guidelines for culturally sensitive mental health practice.* Geelong: Geelong Migrant Resource Centre and Victorian Transcultural Psychiatry Unit.

Klimidis, S., Lewis J., Miletic, T., McKenzie, S., Stolk, Y., & Minas, I.H. (1999) *Mental health service use by ethnic communities in Victoria.* Melbourne: Victorian Transcultural Psychiatry Unit and Centre for Cultural Studies in Health.

Klimidis, S., McKenzie, D.P., Lewis, J., & Minas, I.H. (2002). Continuity of contact with psychiatric services: Immigrant and Australian-born patients. *Social Psychiatry and Psychiatric Epidemiology, 35,* 554–563.

Klimidis, S., & Minas, I.H. (1998). [Collectivism scores for medical students.] Unpublished raw data.

Kline, F., Acosta, F.X., Austin, W., & Johnson, R.G., Jr. (1980). The misunderstood Spanish-speaking patient. *American Journal of Psychiatry, 137,* 1530–1533.

Kluckhohn, C. (1951). Values and value orientations in a theory of action. In T. Parsons & E.A. Shields (Eds.), *Toward a general theory of action.* (pp. 388–433). Cambridge: Harvard University Press.

Kok, L-P. (1988) Race, religion and female suicide attempters in Singapore. *Social Psychiatry and Psychiatric Epidemiology, 23,* 236–239.

Kortmann, F. (1987). Problems in communication in transcultural psychiatry: The self-reporting questionnaire in Ethiopia. *Acta Psychiatrica Scandinavia, 75,* 563–570.

Lambert, T., & Minas, I.H. (1998). Transcultural psychopharmacology and pharmacotherapy. *Australasian Psychiatry, 6,* 61–64.

Landrine, H., & Klonoff, E.A. (1992). Culture and health-related schemas: A review and proposal for interdisciplinary integration. *Health Psychology, 11,* 267–276.

Larson, M.L. (1984). *Meaning based translation: A guide to cross-language equivalence.* New York: University Press of America.

Leff, J. (1973). Culture and the differentiation of emotional states. *British Journal of Psychiatry, 123,* 299–306.

Leff, J. (1988). *Psychiatry around the globe: A Transcultural View.* London: Gaskell.

Lefley, H.P., Sandoval, M.C., & Charles, C. (1998). Traditional healing systems in a multicultural setting. In S.O. Okpaku (Ed.), *Clinical Methods in Transcultural Psychiatry* (pp. 88–110). Washington: American Psychiatric Press.

Leventhal, H., Meyer, D., & Nerenz, D. (1980). The common sense representation of illness danger. In S. Rachman (Ed.), *Contributions to medical psychology* (Vol. 2 pp. 7–30). Oxford: Pergamon Press.

Levine, R.E. ,& Gaw, A.C. (1995). Culture-bound syndromes. *The Psychiatric Clinics of North America, 18,* 523–536.

Lewis, T. (1996) Somali cultural profile — Traditional medical practices. *Ethnomed.* Retrieved 3 April, 1999, from http://healthlinks.washington.edu/clinical/ethnomed/somalicp.html

Lewis-Fernandez, R., & Kleinman, A. (1995) Cultural psychiatry: theoretical, clinical and research issues. *The Psychiatric Clinics of North America, 18,* 433–448.

Lien O. (n.d.) *Vietnamese mental health.* Unpublished paper.

Lien, O., & Rice, P. (1994). The experience of working with Vietnamese patients attending a psychiatric service. In X.T. Nguyen (Ed.), *Vietnamese studies in a multicultural world* (pp. 207–219). Melbourne: Vietnamese Language and Culture Publications.

Lin, K-M. (1996). Cultural influences on the diagnosis of organic and psychotic disorders. In J.E. Mezzich, A. Kleinman, H. Fabrega & D.L. Parron, (Eds.), *Culture and psychiatric diagnosis: A DSM-IV perspective.* (pp. 49–62). Washington: American Psychiatric Press.

Lin, T.Y. (1989). Neurasthenia revisited: Its place in modern psychiatry. *Culture Medicine and Psychiatry, 13,* 105–129.

Littlewood, R. (1996). Cultural comments on culture-bound syndromes: I. In J.E. Mezzich, A. Kleinman, H. Fabrega & D.L. Parron (Eds.), *Culture and psychiatric diagnosis: A DSM-IV perspective.* (pp. 309–312). Washington: American Psychiatric Press.

Littlewood, R., & Lipsedge, M. (1987). The butterfly and the serpent: Culture, psychopathology and biomedicine. *Culture, Medicine and Psychiatry, 11*, 289–335.

Littlewood, R., & Lipsedge, M. (1989). *Aliens and alienists: Ethnic minorities and psychiatry* (2nd ed.). London: Unwin Hyman.

Lock, M. (1987). DSM-III as a culture-bound construct: Commentary on culture-bound syndromes and international disease classifications. *Culture, Medicine and Psychiatry, 11*, 5–42.

Lock, M. (1982). Popular conceptions of mental health in Japan. In A.J. Marsella & G.M. White (Eds.), *Cultural conceptions of mental health and therapy* (pp. 215–233). Dordrecht: Reidel.

Lounsbery, G.C. (1973). *Buddhist meditation in the southern school: Theory and practice for Westerners.* Tucson, Arizona: Omen Press.

Lukoff, D., Lu., F.G., & Turner, R. (1995). Cultural considerations in the assessment and treatment of religious and spiritual problems. *The Psychiatry Clinics of North America, 18*, 467–485.

Luntz, J. (n.d.) *Adolescent NESB mental health project – Background paper No. 3: The Vietnamese understanding of mental health.* Unpublished paper.

Luntz, J. (1998). *Cultural Competence in CAMHS: Report on the usage of child and adolescent mental health services by NESB adolescents and their families.* Melbourne: Austin and Repatriation Medical Centre Child and Adolescent Mental Health Services.

Lutz, C. (1985). Depression and the translation of emotional worlds. In A. Kleinman & B.J. Good (Eds.), *Culture and depression: Studies in the anthropology and cross-cultural psychiatry of affect and disorder.* (pp. 63–100). Berkeley: University of California Press.

McCartney E.S. (1981) Praise and dispraise in folklore. In A. Dundes (Ed.), *The evil eye: A folklore casebook* (pp. 9–38). New York: Garland.

McDonald, B., & Steel Z. (1997). *Immigrants and mental health: An epidemiological analysis.* Sydney: Transcultural Mental Health Centre.

McKenzie, K.J., & Crowcroft, N. (1994). Race, ethnicity, culture, and science *British Medical Journal, 309*, 286–287.

Manson, S.M., Shore, J.H. & Bloom, J.D. (1985). The depressive experience in American Indian communities: A challenge for psychiatric theory and diagnosis. In A. Kleinman & B. Good (Eds.), *Culture and depression: Studies in the anthropology and cross-cultural psychiatry of affect and disorder.* (pp. 331–368). Berkeley: University of California Press.

Marcos, L.R. (1976). Bilinguals in psychotherapy: Language as an emotional barrier. *American Journal of Psychotherapy, 30*, 552–560.

Marcos, L. (1979). Effects of interpreters on the evaluation of psychopathology in non-English speaking patients. *American Journal of Psychiatry, 136,* 171–174.

Marcos, L.R., & Alpert, M. (1976). Strategies and risks in psychotherapy with bilingual patients: The phenomenon of language independence. *American Journal of Psychotherapy, 133,* 1275–1278.

Marcos, L.R., Alpert, M., Urcuyo, L., & Kesselman, M. (1973). The effect of interview language on the evaluation of psychopathology in Spanish-American schizophrenic patients. *American Journal of Psychiatry, 130,* 549–553.

Marcos, L.R., Urcuyo, L., Kesselman, M., Alpert, M. (1973) The language barrier in evaluating Spanish-American patients. *Archives of General Psychiatry, 29,* 655–659.

Markus, H.R., & Kitayama, S. (1991). Culture and the self: Implications for cognition, emotion and motivation. *Psychological Review, 98,* 224–253.

Markus, H.R., Mullaly, P.R. & Kitayama, S. (1997). Selfways: Diversity in modes of cultural participation. In U. Neisser & D. Jopling (Eds.), *The conceptual self in context.* (pp. 13–60). New York: Cambridge University Press.

Mezzich, J.E., Kleinman, A., Fabrega, H., & Parron, D.L. (1996). Introduction. *Culture and psychiatric diagnosis: A DSM-IV perspective.* (pp. xvii–xxiii). Washington: American Psychiatric Press.

Minas, I.H. (1990). Mental health in a culturally diverse society. In J. Reid & P. Trompf (Eds.), *The health of immigrant Australia: A social perspective* (pp. 250–287). Sydney: Harcourt Brace Jovanovich.

Minas, I.H. (1991). Psychiatric services research in a multicultural society. In I.H. Minas (Ed.), *Cultural diversity and mental health* (pp. 35–51). Melbourne: Royal Australian and New Zealand College of Psychiatrists and Victorian Transcultural Psychiatry Unit.

Minas, I.H. (1996a). *A transcultural guide for mental health clinicians.* Melbourne: Victorian Transcultural Psychiatry Unit.

Minas, I.H. (1996b). *Transcultural psychiatry. Current Opinion in psychiatry, 9,* 144–148.

Minas, I.H. (1998) Cultural diversity: Ethics and practice. *Chiron, 4,* 8–10.

Minas, I.H., & Evert, H. (n.d.). *Vietnamese community mental health profile.* Melbourne: Victorian Transcultural Psychiatry Unit.

Minas, I.H., Lambert, T.J.R., Kostov, S., & Boranga, G. (1996). *Mental health services for NESB immigrants: Transforming policy into practice.* Canberra: Australian Government Publishing Service.

Minas, I.H., Read, P., & Klimidis, S. (1999, October). *Individualism/collectivism and suicide: Cross-national trends.* Poster session presented at the Australian Transcultural Mental Health Network Conference, Melbourne.

Murdock, G.P., Wilson, S.F., & Frederick, V. (1980). World distribution of theories of illness. *Transcultural Psychiatric Research Review, 17,* 37–64.

Murdock, G.P., Wilson, S.F., & Frederick, V. (1978). World distribution of theories of illness. *Ethnology, 17,* 449–470.

Mugoci, A. (1981). The evil eye in Roumania and its antidotes. In A. Dundes (Ed.), *The evil eye: A folklore casebook* (pp. 124–130). New York: Garland.

Myers, H.F., Wohlford, P., Guzman, L.P., & Echemendia, R.J. (1991) *Ethnic minority perspectives on clinical training and services in psychology.* Washington: American Psychological Association.

Neisser U. (1966). *Cognitive psychology.* New York: Appleton-Century-Crofts.

Ng, C.H. (1997). The stigma of mental illness in Asian cultures. *Australian and New Zealand Journal of Psychiatry, 31,* 382–390.

Obeyesekere, G. (1985). Depression, Buddhism, and the work of culture in Sri Lanka. In A. Kleinman & B. Good (Eds.), *Culture and depression: Studies in the anthropology and cross-cultural psychiatry of affect and disorder* (pp. 134–152). Berkeley: University of California Press.

Oquendo, M.A. (1996). Psychiatric evaluation and psychotherapy in the patient's second language. *Psychiatric Services, 47,* 614–618.

Pardy, M. (1995). *"Speaking of speaking": Experiences of women and interpreting.* Fitzroy, Victoria: Clearing House on Migration Issues.

Patel, V., Musara, T., Butau, T., Maramba, P., & Fuyane, S. (1995). Concepts of mental illness and medical pluralism in Harare. *Psychological Medicine, 25,* 485–493.

Patel, V., & Winston, M. (1994). Universality of mental illness revisited: Assumptions, artefacts and new directions. *British Journal of Psychiatry, 165,* 437–440.

Phan, T., & Silove, S. (1997). The influence of culture on psychiatric assessment: The Vietnamese refugee. *Psychiatric Services, 48,* 86–90.

Pilowsky, I. (1997). *Abnormal illness behaviour.* New York: John Wiley.

Pilowsky, I., & Spence, N.D. (1977). Ethnicity and illness behaviour. *Psychological Medicine, 7,* 447–452.

Prince, R. (1985). The concept of culture-bound syndromes: Anorexia nervosa and brain-fag. *Social Science and Medicine, 21,* 197–203.

Ragurum, R., Weiss, M.G., Channabasavanna, S.M., & Devins, G.M. (1996). Stigma, depression ,and somatization in South India. *American Journal of Psychiatry, 153,* 1043–1049.

Robbins, J.M., & Kirmayer, L.J. (1991). Cognitive and social factors in somatization. In L.J. Kirmayer & J.M. Robbins (Eds.), *Current concepts of somatization: Research and clinical perspectives* (pp. 107–141). Washington: American Psychiatric Press.

Rogler, L.H. (1993). Culture in psychiatric diagnosis: An issue of scientific accuracy. *Psychiatry, 56,* 324–327.

Rotem, O. (1996). Buddhism. In C. Scott Littleton (Ed.), *The sacred East: Hinduism, Buddhism, Confucianism, Daoism, Shinto* (pp. 54–91). Melbourne: Cardigan Street Publishers.

Royal Park Corporation. (1994). *Ethnic health audit.* Melbourne: Royal Park Hospital.

Sang, D. (1996). Health and illness in the Vietnamese community in Western Australia. In I.H. Minas (Ed.), *Recent developments in mental health* (pp. 152–153). Proceedings of a collaborative workshop between Vietnam, Australia and New Zealand, Hanoi. Melbourne: Centre for Cultural Studies in Health, University of Melbourne.

Sartorius, N., Jablensky, A., Gulbinat, W., & Ernberg, G. (1980). Preliminary communication. WHO collaborative study: Assessment of depressive disorders. *Psychological Medicine, 10,* 743–749.

Schwartz, S.H., & Bilsky, W. (1987). Toward a universal psychological structure of human values. *Journal of Personality and Social Psychology, 53,* 550–562.

Schreiber, S. (1995). Migration, traumatic bereavement and transcultural aspects of psychological healing: Loss and grief of a refugee woman from Begameder County in Ethiopia. *British Journal of Medical Psychology, 68,* 135–142.

Scott Littleton, C. (1996). *The sacred East: Hinduism, Buddhism, Confucianism, Daoism, Shinto.* Melbourne: Cardigan Street Publishers.

Senior, P.A., & Bhopal, R. (1994). Ethnicity as a key variable in epidemiological research. *British Medical Journal, 309,* 327–330.

Sharp, L. (1994). Exorcists, psychiatrists, and the problems of possession in North-West Madagascar. *Social Science and Medicine, 38,* 525–542.

Shweder, R.A. (1985). Menstrual pollution, soul loss, and the comparative study of emotions. In A. Kleinman & B.J. Good (Eds.), *Culture and depression: Studies in the anthropology and cross-cultural psychiatry of affect and disorder* (pp. 182–215). Berkeley: University of California Press.

Shweder, R.A., & Bourne, E.J. (1982). Does the concept of the person vary cross-culturally? In A.J. Marsella & G.M. White (Eds.), *Cultural conceptions of mental health and therapy* (pp. 97–137). Dordrecht: Reidel.

Sidel, R. (1975) Mental diseases in China and their treatment. In T.J. Scheff (Ed.), *Labelling madness* (pp. 119–134). Englewood Cliff, NJ: Prentice-Hall.

Smith, P.B., & Bond, M.H. (1993). *Social psychology across cultures: Analysis and perspectives.* New York: Harvester Wheatsheaf.

Stein, D.J. (1993). Cross-cultural psychiatry and the DSM-IV. *Comprehensive Psychiatry, 34,* 322–329.

Stolk, Y. (1996) *Access to psychiatric services by people of non-English speaking background in the Western Metropolitan Region of Melbourne.* Volumes 1 & 2. Melbourne: Victorian Transcultural Psychiatry Unit.

Stolk, Y. (2002). *Development and evaluation of a training program in crosscultural psychiatric assessment.* Doctoral dissertation in preparation, Centre for International Mental Health, University of Melbourne.

Strongman, K.T., & Strongman, L. (1996). Maori emotion. In R. Harre & W.G. Parrot (Eds.), *The emotions: Social, cultural and biological dimensions* (pp. 200–203). London: Sage Publications.

Sue, D.W., Bernier, Y., Durran, A., Feinberg, L., Pedersen, P.B., Smith, E.J., & Vasquez-Nuttal, E. (1982). Position paper: Cross-cultural counselling competencies. *Counselling Psychologist, 10,* 45–52.

Sue, D., & Sue, S. (1987). Cultural factors in the clinical assessment of Asian Americans. *Journal of Consulting and Clinical Psychology, 55,* 479–487.

Sue, S., & Zane, N. (1987). The role of culture and cultural techniques in psychotherapy: A critique and reformulation. *American Psychologist, 42,* 37–45.

Swartz, L. (1998). *Culture and mental health: A Southern African view.* Cape Town: Oxford University Press.

Triandis, H.C. (1990). Theoretical concepts that are applicable to the analysis of ethnocentrism. In R.W. Brislin (Ed.), *Applied cross-cultural psychology* (pp. 34–55). London: Sage.

Tseng, W.S. (1999). Culture and psychotherapy: Review and practical guidelines. *Transcultural Psychiatry, 36,* 131–179.

Turk, D.C., Rudy, T.E., & Salovey, P. (1986). Implicit models of illness. *Journal of Behavioral Medicine, 9,* 453–474.

Walter, G., & Rey, J.M. (1999). The relevance of herbal treatments for psychiatric practice. *Australian and New Zealand Journal of Psychiatry, 33,* 482–489.

Weber, M. (1963). *The sociology of religion.* Boston: Beacon Press.

Weiss, C.I. (1992). Controlling domestic life and mental illness: Spiritual and aftercare resources used by Dominican New Yorkers. *Culture Medicine and Psychiatry, 16,* 237–271.

Wessells, M. (1997). Reintegrating Africa's child soldiers: An In-Psych interview. *In-Psych, June,* 14–16.

Westermeyer, J. (1985). Psychiatric diagnosis across cultural boundaries. *American Journal of Psychiatry, 142,* 798–805.

Westermeyer, J. (1987) Cultural factors in clinical assessment. *Journal of Consulting and Clinical Psychology, 55,* 471–478.

Westermeyer, J., Janca, A., & Sartorius, N. (1993). *A sociocultural lexicon for psychiatry (to accompany ICD-10). Draft copy.* Geneva: World Health Organization, Mental Health Division.

Westermeyer, J., & Janca, A. (1997). Language, culture and psychopathology: Conceptual and methodological issues. *Transcultural Psychiatry, 34,* 291–311.

White, G.M. (1982). The ethnographic study of cultural knowledge of "mental disorder". In A.J. Marsella & G.M. White (Eds.), *Cultural conceptions of mental health and therapy* (pp. 69–95). Dordrecht: Reidel.

Wierzbicka, A. (1992). Talking about emotions: Semantics, culture and cognition. *Cognition and Emotion, 6,* 285–319.

Winfrey, L.P.L., & Goldfried, M.R. (1986). Information processing and the human change process. In R.E. Ingram (Ed.), *Information processing approaches in clinical psychology* (pp. 241–258). Orlando: Academic Press.

Woodburne, A.S. (1981) The evil eye in South Indian folklore. In A. Dundes (Ed.), *The evil eye: A folklore casebook* (pp. 55–65). New York: Garland.

World Health Organization. (1992). *International statistical classification of diseases and related health problems* (10th rev.). Geneva: Author.

Young, A. (1976). Internalising and externalising medical belief systems: An Ethiopian example. *Social Science and Medicine, 10,* 147–156.

Young, B., & Papadatou, D. (1997). Childhood, death and bereavement across cultures. In C.M. Parkes, P. Laungani & B. Young (Eds.), *Death and bereavement across cultures* (pp. 191–205). London: Routledge.

Zealberg, J.J., Hardesty, S.J., & Tyson, S.C. (1998). Emergency psychiatry: Mental health clinicians' role in responding to critical incidents in the community. *Psychiatric Services, 49,* 301–303.

Ziguras, S., Stuart, G., Klimidis, S., Minas, H., Lewis, J., Pennella, J., & Jackson, A. (2000). *Evaluation of the Bilingual Case Management Program.* Melbourne: Victorian Transcultural Psychiatry Unit.

Zvirblis, M., & Dixon, C. (1993). *The Hmong woman: A case study.* Paper presented at Australia's First International Psychiatric Nursing Conference, Melbourne.

Index

www.ingramcontent.com/pod-product-compliance
Ingram Content Group Australia Pty Ltd
76 Discovery Rd, Dandenong South VIC 3175, AU
AUHW011250130325
408272AU00010B/36

9 781875 378401